Curing the Patient, Not the Disease

"There are very few incurable diseases," said the old man, "but there are many incurable patients. These are people who are not able or willing to allow themselves to be healed."

"But surely everybody wants to be healthy?" argued the young man.

"In their conscious mind, perhaps so, but in their subconscious mind, sometimes, it is not so. If everybody wanted to be healthy, would they partake of unhealthy practices? Would they knowingly destroy their health by smoking cigarettes, drinking much alcohol, and eating junk foods?"

"I see your point," said the young man.

"When these people get sick, they refuse to change their lifestyles and instead prefer to cling on to their health-destroying habits until the damage cannot be reversed. These people are incurable from the very start of their illness. It is not the illness itself which is incurable, it is people who make themselves incurable. These people are not interested in building health, only in avoiding pain and disease."

BY ADAM J. JACKSON

The Secrets of Abundant Happiness
*The Secrets of Abundant Wealth**
*The Secrets of Abundant Love**

*To be published by HarperPaperbacks

The TEN SECRETS *of* ABUNDANT HEALTH

*A Modern Parable of Wisdom
and Health That Will Change
Your Life*

ADAM J. JACKSON

HarperPaperbacks
A Division of HarperCollinsPublishers

HarperPaperbacks *A Division of* HarperCollins*Publishers*
10 East 53rd Street, New York, N.Y. 10022

A trade paperback edition of this book was published in 1996 in Great Britain by Thorsons, an imprint of HarperCollins*Publishers*.

Cover and interior illustrations by Joan Perrin Falquet

First HarperPaperbacks printing: August 1996

Printed in the United States of America

HarperPaperbacks and colophon are trademarks of HarperCollins*Publishers*

❖ 10 9 8 7 6 5 4 3 2 1

*This book is dedicated to the memory of
Dr. Emil Just, to his beautiful wife, Edith,
and to Fred Kurgen—three very special people
who first inspired and guided me in my work—
with love and gratitude.*

Contents

Acknowledgments

I would like to thank all those people who have helped me in my work and in the writing of this book. I am particularly grateful to:

My literary agent, Sara Menguc, and her assistant, Georgia Glover, for all their efforts and work on my behalf.

Everyone at Thorsons, but especially Erica Smith for her enthusiasm and constructive comments throughout the writing of the book, and Fiona Brown who edited the manuscript.

My mother, who always encouraged me to write, and remains a constant source of inspiration and love to me; my father for his encouragement, guidance, and help in all my work, and all of my family and friends for their love.

And finally, to Karen—my wife, my best friend, and my most candid editor. Words cannot express my love for the one person who has always had faith in me and believed in my work.

Introduction

> The doctor of the future will give no medicine,
> but will instead interest his patients in the care
> of the human frame, in diet, and in the cause
> and prevention of disease.
>
> —*Thomas Edison*

We all desire good health, but why is it that so few people are healthy? Why is it that despite the advances of modern medicine, the growth of sales in drugs, and the vast array of nutritional supplements, afflictions such as cancer, heart disease, diabetes, asthma, and nervous disorders have become more prevalent with each passing decade? Could it be that we are searching for health in the wrong places?

I believe that we are all responsible for our own health and the health of our children, and that we all have the power to create not just health, but Abundant Health in our lives. Abundant Health is not just a state of being free from any identifiable disease—many people have no diagnosed illness but still feel continually tired, run down, and listless—it is rather a state of abundant well-being, energy, and vitality that enables us to live our lives to the full. Unlike most other parables, all of the characters in this book are based upon real people (with the exception of the old Chinese man who is based upon a composite of several old wise men and women I have met). Their names have, of course, been changed, but they all overcame their diseases and found health as recorded in each chapter. It is my hope that their stories will inspire you to take action so that you too may experience the blessing of Abundant Health in your own life.

Adam J. Jackson
Hertfordshire
March 1995

The
TEN
SECRETS
of
ABUNDANT
HEALTH

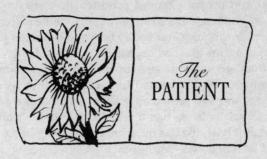

The
PATIENT

The young man's face was pale as he left the doctor's surgery. His hand trembled as he closed the door behind him and his eyes became more puffy and glazed with each step. He stared vacantly ahead, his mind oblivious to all around him, as he walked down the corridor and into the reception area of the university clinic. Suddenly he felt weak, the room began spinning, and it was all he could do to reach out to the nearest chair and haul himself onto it.

The rain beat heavily against the large windows next to the entrance. One bitter question kept pounding in his mind, a question that many people ask when facing such a crisis: "Why me?"

He was not aware that questions focusing on the

past and on pain cannot produce answers for the future. Such questions can only lead to more suffering and more anguish and finally he could no longer hold back the tears that had been welling up inside him.

It all seemed to have happened so quickly, almost overnight. He had settled in well to his first year at college and had passed all his exams with top grades. By all accounts, he had a wonderful future ahead of him. But now, the one most important thing in his life had let him down—his health.

Health is supposedly our most prized possession but it is something we all too often take for granted and consequently neglect. Many people take greater care of their cars than they do of their own bodies, and the young man was no exception.

But health cannot be neglected forever. Sooner or later a day arrives when we are forced to sit up and think again and this was one such day for the young man. Now all he could hear were the doctor's parting words: "Nothing can be done ... I'm sorry. There is no cure."

All of a sudden his life had been turned upside down and would never be the same again.

And so, in a corner of the college vestibule, the young man sat with his head in his hands. Desperate, frightened, and alone, he did something that he had not done since his childhood ... he prayed. But this was no ordinary prayer, it was a prayer from the very depths of his heart, "Oh, God, please help me. Please show me the way."

Prayer brings mysterious power—an intangible energy connecting the spirit with a higher power; a power that, if correctly channeled, will overcome any problem and remedy any illness. Communication of the mind and spirit to a divine force brings peace, a calmness to transcend all distress, and very often, if the prayer is sincere and the faith strong, a miracle happens . . . the prayer is answered.

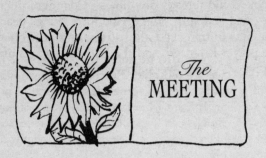

The
MEETING

"You look troubled. Can I help you?"

The young man turned to find an elderly Chinese gentleman standing next to him. He was a small, unassuming man with dark brown eyes and a totally bald head save for the pure white hair around the sides.

"I'll be all right, thank you," he whispered.

The old man sat down anyway.

"You know," he said, "in my country we believe every problem brings with it a gift."

"There is no gift in my problem," mumbled the young man.

"Oh, I assure you that there is," replied his new

4

companion. "Sometimes it is difficult to see, but it is always there. Even in sickness."

The young man was startled. What did the old man mean? Why did he refer to "sickness"? He turned to face the old man. He could not remember meeting him before but something about him was very familiar. It wasn't his face. He would not have forgotten his face. It was a kind, gentle face with warm eyes. Perhaps it was his voice, but then again, he felt sure he would have remembered such a soft oriental accent. No, he didn't know what it was but the old man seemed very familiar to him. He could only assume that the old man was one of the new lecturers on sabbatical from abroad.

"What 'gift' can there possibly be in sickness?" muttered the young man.

"Suffering often brings forth greater joys. Just as the darkness of night prepares the way for the dawn and out of the pain of childbirth is born Nature's greatest miracle, it is through sickness that we receive the gift of Abundant Health."

The young man was confused. "How could sickness produce health?" he thought, but before he had time to ask, the old man continued.

"Sickness is simply the body's way of healing itself. When you have a cold or flu, it is really an indication of your body fighting off invading germs. When you have a stomachache, your body is telling you something you have eaten or done has upset it. Even when you have a backache, it is often just your body's way of telling you that a muscle is strained and is in need of rest.

"You see, sickness, pain, and disease are really our friends: they are God's messengers telling us when something is wrong and needs to be fixed. Pain is a voice that calls out to help us."

"Well, it's one 'voice' I could do without," interjected the young man.

"Ah, but could you?" asked the old man. "Imagine what your life would be like if you could not feel any pain. You would be dead before you knew it. One day you could be sitting next to an open fire and look down to find that your arm has been burned to a stub, all because you could not hear pain's voice telling you to move your arm away.

"Most people believe, like you, that pain is their worst enemy and so they try to kill it or silence its voice by using medications. But killing the pain alone never solves the problem. If the *cause* of a disease is not removed, the disease will always get worse. In the end, stronger and stronger medications are needed to kill the pain and those drugs often bring more problems."

The young man thought about his own experience. It was certainly true that he had developed more symptoms after he had started taking the medications his doctor had originally prescribed.

"But what if a disease is incurable?" he urged. "Where is the blessing then?"

"There are very few incurable diseases," said the old man, "but there are many incurable patients. These are people who are not able or willing to allow themselves to be healed."

"But surely everybody wants to be healthy?" argued the young man.

"In their conscious mind, perhaps so, but in their subconscious mind, sometimes, it is not so. If everybody wanted to be healthy, would they partake of unhealthy practices? Would they knowingly destroy their health by smoking cigarettes, drinking much alcohol, and eating junk foods?"

"I see your point," said the young man.

"When these people get sick, they refuse to change their lifestyles and instead prefer to cling on to their health-destroying habits until the damage cannot be reversed. These people are incurable from the very start of their illness, do you see? It is not the illness itself which is incurable, it is people who make themselves incurable. These people are not interested in building health, only in avoiding pain and disease."

"But surely health is more complicated than that?" argued the young man.

"Not really. In fact it is very simple. Why do you think people become ill in the first place?" asked the old man.

"I don't know, these things just happen, don't they? That's what my doctor said. I suppose it's fate or bad luck."

"Really? Do you not think that there may be a reason for an illness?"

"I'm not sure."

The old man looked at the young man and said, "Can you think of one thing that happens in Nature without something causing it to happen? Look at the rain outside, does it fall by accident? Do the clouds just happen to form?"

The old man continued, 'There are laws in Nature. Water begins to boil at 100 degrees centigrade, not at 99 or 101, but exactly 100. Similarly, it freezes at exactly 0 degrees centigrade."

The old man took a coin out of his pocket and said, "If I let go of this coin, what will happen?"

"It will drop to the ground," said the young man.

"Why will it fall? By some chance or luck?"

"No, of course not, it falls because it is heavier than air. It's the law of gravity," said the young man.

"Exactly," said the old man, "the law of gravity which is just one of the many laws of Nature. Do you see, nothing happens in the universe by chance. Health and disease are not matters of luck. Far from it; health is simply the inevitable result of living in harmony with the laws of Nature and all disease is the inevitable result of living contrary to the laws of Nature.

"If a person smokes, is it likely he will have healthy lungs?"

"No, of course not," answered the young man.

"If people eat junk food, is it likely they will be well nourished?"

"No, I see what you mean," said the young man, "but what about germs and viruses? They cause disease but what do they have to do with the way we live?"

"Germs are like rats," explained the old man, "they accumulate only in unhealthy environments. The one way to guarantee that you'll get rats in your house is by not cleaning it. If you keep your house clean, rats will not be attracted because they have nothing to feed off."

"But sometimes people can catch a germ," argued the young man.

"Germs do not, by themselves, *cause* disease, otherwise everybody who had a disease would also have the offending germ in their bloodstream and everybody who had the germ in their bloodstream would also have the disease. Neither is true. Just as rats feed off waste matter accumulated in and around the home, germs feed off waste matter in and around the body. And, just as rats cannot survive in a clean environment because there is nothing for them to feed off, so too germs cannot survive in a healthy bloodstream.

"People are far too concerned about germs and far too little concerned about the environments that *attract* germs. No matter how much they try, they can never be free of rats until they get rid of the things the rats feed off.

"This is why health can only be created and disease can only be overcome through healthy living. All health and healing must begin by changing one's lifestyle to suit the laws of Nature."

"It makes sense but it seems too simple," said the young man.

The old man smiled. "That's because it *is* simple. It is so simple and yet for many people so difficult to understand. There are fixed and immutable laws in Nature that will, if followed, create health and, just as surely, if transgressed, produce disease."

The young man could see that the old man had a point but he was not sure where the logic in his argument was leading.

"Let me explain," said the old man. "All disease is only 'dis-ease' inside the body, yes?"

"Yes."

"All dis-ease is caused by something, yes?"

"Yes, I suppose so."

"Then to eliminate dis-ease and create 'ease' (or health), it is necessary to remove the *cause* of the disease, yes?"

The young man nodded in partial agreement.

The old man continued. "Take a look at that gentleman over there," he said, pointing to a man sitting alone at the end of the row of chairs. "He began 10 years ago suffering a few migraine headaches every week. The migraines were actually being caused by his diet. He ate lots of chocolate, cheese, and meat, and he drank several large glasses of alcohol every day. He could have removed the cause of his migraines by changing his diet. But instead, he chose to take medications that suppressed his pain.

"After a year or so, he needed stronger medications, but the new medications actually caused high blood pressure and so he was given more medications to control the high blood pressure. Today he has a disease called atherosclerosis—hardening of the arteries—which has endangered his heart and completely changed his quality of life. He has to take tablets every day, his heart is so weak that he cannot run or walk briskly, and he requires surgery to fit a pacemaker to activate his heart. On top of it all, he still gets migraines, only much more frequently. His condition has been created because he chose to kill his initial pain instead of removing the cause of his problem.

"You see, true healing never comes from tablets or potions. Health is never found in a bottle or in a surgeon's knife. Of course, I do not say that certain medicines and methods of surgery do not have their place—in crisis situations they can save lives—but they can never by themselves *create* health. Nothing outside the body can heal or create health."

"But if medicines do not create health, what does?" asked the young man.

"Well, let's see," said the old man. "Imagine, for a moment, you are hammering a picture pin in a wall, and quite by accident you miss the pin and bruise your thumb. Will it get better?"

"Yes, of course," said the young man.

"Without any tablets or ointments the thumb will heal, yes?"

The young man nodded.

"But why?" asked the old man.

"It just does," said the young man.

"Ah! You see? 'It just does.' Because your body has a healing force within it and this heals all ailments," said the old man. "But what would happen if you went back to the hammering the next day and you hit your thumb again, and the following day yet again, and every other day you went right back and hit your thumb? And hit it again and again and again. Would it get better?"

"Not if I kept banging it, no."

"Of course, because you would not have removed the cause of the pain and your body's healing force cannot work until you have removed the cause of the problem. But once you stop hitting your thumb it will heal itself because there is a wonderful healing force inside you.

"The same thing happens throughout Nature; when a tree branch is lopped the tree bleeds and then repairs itself. Everyone is blessed with a healing force that will always, when given the proper conditions, heal the body of all dis-eases if only we give it the right conditions.

"All day, every day, many people are banging little hammers inside their bodies through poor living habits and creating more and more dis-ease. To eliminate the dis-ease all they need to do is stop banging. Remove the cause of the illness and you remove the illness itself.

"In this world, my friend, you can only reap that which you have sown. It is the law of cause and effect. You are and always have been in control of your destiny. This is why the path to health begins with the understanding that you have created your own state of health or disease, and therefore you have the power to change it.

"Every person has the ability not only to heal himself but also to create Abundant Health . . . by changing his lifestyle. All it takes is the awareness of the Laws of Nature and an acceptance that you are responsible for your own state of health. No one else is responsible—doctors, parents, teachers, therapists—none of them are responsible for your health. The moment you accept responsibility for your own health is the moment you will begin to conquer disease and create Abundant Health in your life."

Now it was all beginning to make sense to the young man. He had never considered that his health was created or destroyed by his own actions. Consequently he had never bothered to learn what his body needed to stay healthy.

The young man took a close look at the old man and for the first time noticed that this was no ordinary old man. Old men, he thought, were supposed to be bent over, frail, and weak. Old men were meant to be ill. Yet this particular old man held himself so erect and strong. In fact, he had quite a striking appearance for a man of his age. His skin seemed to glow and his eyes were bright, almost sparkling. The young man had simply never seen such vibrant energy in anyone he had ever met before, let alone such an elderly man. If the way he looked was anything to go by, there must be some truth in what he was saying.

"Remember," said the old man, "we all have the power to conquer disease and create Abundant Health in our lives. Abundant Health is much more than the mere absence of disease. It is energy, power, a zest for living and the joy of life.

"All you have to do is live in harmony with the laws of Nature. Everything in the universe is governed by precise laws . . . including your health. These laws contain the secrets which have the power to conquer all disease and create Abundant Health in our lives."

"But what are these secrets?" asked the young man.

"They are the secrets of Abundant Health," answered the old man as he wrote out a list of 10 names and 10 telephone numbers on a piece of paper. "Contact each of these people in turn and they will teach you what you wish to learn. They have all acquired and mastered the secrets of Abundant Health.

"But remember what I am about to say, for in matters of health and disease, nothing is more simple or more important:

"For every symptom there is a cause. Therefore remove the cause and you will remove the symptom. In this light, every ailment has a remedy just as every problem has a solution.

"It is promised in the Bible, 'Those who ask shall be given, for those who knock, the door shall be opened, and those who seek, shall find.' Therefore, seek your health with all your heart and you will surely find it."

With those words the old man handed the piece of paper to the young man. The young man examined the list of 10 names for only a few seconds, but when he turned to face the old man, he found the chair beside him empty. The old man had gone as quickly as he had first appeared.

There was so much the young man wanted to ask, so many questions. He went straight to the administrator's office and asked who the new Chinese lecturer was and where he might be found.

"Who are you talking about?" asked the administrator. "There are no new Chinese lecturers. And there are no new Japanese or Taiwanese lecturers either."

"Are you sure?" persisted the young man.

"Of course I'm sure. In fact, the only Asian lecturer on our staff is Mrs. Chang in the Maths department. And she has been with us for five years now."

The young man was perplexed. Who was the old man? Where had he come from? Even more importantly, could it really be possible that the old man was right? Did laws of Health really exist? It had all happened so fast it could have been a dream, the old man a figment of his imagination. But then he looked down and he knew that the old man was real, the meeting had been no dream. The proof was in his hands—a piece of paper containing a list of 10 names.

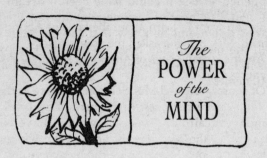

The
POWER
of the
MIND

The first name on the young man's list was a woman by the name of Karen Selsdon. Wasting no time, he telephoned her the minute he returned home from college. He explained his story to her and suddenly she seemed to be as enthusiastic to meet him as he was to meet her. They agreed to meet at 3 P.M. the following day.

All through the morning, the young man could not keep his thoughts from wondering what the first meeting would bring, but by 3 P.M. he was finally sitting in front of his first teacher. Mrs. Selsdon was married with two small children and she was also a clinical psychologist. The young man could not think why psychology could have anything to do with his health. After all, as far as he knew he was not psychologically disturbed.

"So you want to learn about the laws of Abundant Health?" Mrs. Selsdon asked the young man.

"Are there really laws of Abundant Health?" asked the young man.

"Of course," replied Mrs. Selsdon, "as sure as there are laws governing all of Nature. The laws of Abundant Health are precise laws that have been with us since the beginning of time. When we know the laws and how they work we can overcome any illness and create a level of health that most people only dream about.

"There are many facets that go toward creating health but the one in which I am most qualified and the one that has certainly had the greatest impact in my life is the power of the mind. People often mistakenly believe that the mind only affects our emotions and mental health but the truth is, the mind is where all health originates—emotional and physical. And all disease, for that matter."

"Why is the mind so important?" asked the young man.

"Because your mind controls your body. You can see the power of the mind every day. When people get embarrassed their faces flush, when they are frightened their faces turn pale and, when they get nervous, their palms often become sweaty and their knees shake. All these are examples of the many ways our mind can affect our body.

"Let me show you something," she said. "Close your eyes for a moment and try to imagine a lemon."

The young man sat back in his chair and shut his eyes. "Okay, I see a lemon," he said.

"Now imagine that you are taking a big bite right into that lemon."

The young man's face grimaced and he could feel his teeth go on edge just as if he had actually taken a bite from a real lemon.

"You see how powerful your mind is," Mrs. Selsdon said. "All you did was imagine a lemon and your body reacted as if it was the real thing. That is the power of the mind. You see, your mind controls your thoughts and your thoughts control everything in your body. In exactly the same way as we can use the power of our mind to make our mouth salivate, we can use it to boost our immune system by increasing the production of our white blood cells, and we can also use that same power to relieve pain, clear skin disorders, and even to help cure many diseases including cancer.

"When I first learned of it I was as skeptical as you look," she said. "But believe me, the power of my mind helped save my life. Ten years ago I had a malignant tumor in my brain. I was told by my doctor that the tumor was so advanced that it was too dangerous even to operate. Nothing could be done and I was given less than a year to live. I was devastated as you might imagine and I really thought I was going to die. But as you can see I survived."

"What happened?" the young man interjected.

"I met a man who helped save my life. A little old Chinese man!"

The young man felt a tingle go through his spine. Had he thought about it, he would have realized this was just another example of how his mind could affect his body.

"I met him in the city library," continued Mrs. Selsdon. "At the time, I was an assistant librarian working in the reference section and one day he came in and asked for a copy of a book on creative visualization and another on the healing power of the mind.

"We didn't have those books in stock and so I had to order them. Usually an order for books would take a week or so to arrive but on this occasion they were on my desk the following morning. The titles intrigued me and so I read them myself. The essence of the books, one of which was written by a doctor, was that most illnesses could be healed by the power of the mind. Many cases were recorded including patients with cancerous tumors who had survived and got rid of their cancers simply by using the power of their minds. It seemed incredible and so I decided to try the suggested techniques myself."

"What exactly did you do?" asked the young man, eager to find out.

"Well, firstly, I did something called 'creative visualization.' This is a technique in which you create healing images in your mind. I tried to picture the tumor in my head and I imagined it was being eaten by little sharks. Every morning and evening I would lie down or sit in a comfortable chair for fifteen minutes or so and imagine the tumor being eaten up. And, at the end of each session I really did feel better and stronger."

"Really?" said the young man.

"Yes. Really. You can try it for yourself. In fact, why not do a quick one here and now. Close your eyes and take a few deep breaths . . . That's good . . . Now see your health problem in your mind . . . now imagine it being killed off. You can use any images you want. Guns, spacemen, cowboys and Indians, whatever takes your fancy. You can even imagine your problem dissolving away like a block of ice melting in the sun. The images you use don't matter, the important thing is to imagine your body healing."

The young man imagined powerful rocket ships inside him shooting at their target and he then imagined himself looking and feeling healthy and strong. After a few minutes Mrs. Selsdon told him to stop.

"How do you feel now?" she asked.

"Would you believe it?" he exclaimed. "It is very relaxing and I feel like I've got a little more energy than before."

"Good. That's how you should feel. Now imagine how you would feel if you did this exercise for a little bit longer, say 15–20 minutes, two or three times every day."

"I see what you mean," said the young man.

"There is one other very important technique I used to fully utilize the power of my mind, called 'healing affirmations,'" said Mrs. Selsdon.

"I'm sorry, you've lost me there. What are 'healing affirmations'?" asked the young man.

"An affirmation is very simply a statement that you choose to 'affirm' to yourself. That is, you say it over and over either aloud or in your mind. Saying it aloud is more effective."

"How does it work?" asked the young man.

"Well, when you repeat something often enough, it becomes imprinted in your mind. You can't help but imagine whatever you say. For instance, if I tell you not to think of pink elephants wearing purple and white polka-dot tutus, what picture goes through your mind?"

The young man instantly saw a picture in his head of pink elephants wearing purple and white polka-dot tutus.

"I see what you mean," he said. "I can't *not* think of them. So, what you are saying is that by repeating a healing affirmation over and over, my mind cannot avoid focusing on healing and health."

"Exactly," replied Mrs. Selsdon. "Healing affirmations are simply positive healing statements which will, if repeated regularly each day, become imprinted in your mind. Even if at first you don't believe the affirmation you are saying, it will eventually become part of your subconscious, and once it is in your subconscious it will become part of your body. Therefore, the more frequently the affirmation is repeated, the quicker and more effective it will be.

"The value of healing affirmations was first discovered by Dr. Emil Coué in the last century. He would ask his patients to say as often as they could—morning, noon, and night, whenever and wherever possible—a very simple but very effective statement: 'Every day, in every way, I am getting better and better.'

"And do you know, most of the patients who followed his advice did get better!"

"So you overcame your illness," asked the young man, "using healing visualizations and affirmations?"

"Well, I did do other things too. I completely changed my lifestyle. I changed my diet, I exercised regularly, I did deep breathing exercises, and I even learned to laugh and take life less seriously, all of which helped me. You will learn about these things I'm sure in due course from people better qualified than I. But I can assure you that a vital part in my recovery was using the power of my mind. I was so impressed with the effect that, a year later, after I was fully recovered and the tumor had disappeared, I went back to college and studied psychology to learn more about how and why it worked so that I could help other people.

"And if there is one thing I have learned it is this: the foundation of health and disease is the mind. It is really an extremely powerful force that directs our actions and behavior and controls every organ and every cell inside your body. Let me show you something." The woman put a cassette into a video recorder and pressed the play button. "Everything you will see I witnessed with my own eyes. I actually did some of the filming," she said.

The film that came onto the screen was absolutely incredible. It began with people, lots of different people, walking barefoot across red hot coals. The young man recognized Mrs. Selsdon herself on the film and watched spellbound as she walked over the coals.

"This is called the firewalk experience. Over 100 people walked completely barefoot across burning coals heated to over 1,000 centigrade, yet no one felt any pain and not one person had so much as a blister."

"That's impossible!" exclaimed the young man.

"Very little is impossible in this world, believe me," she said with a smile.

"But how did those people do it?"

"The power of the mind!"

The film continued to another scene. This time there was one woman lying in a hospital bed. A man was talking to her and within a moment she was lying very still. A group of people wearing surgical masks and overalls entered the room.

"What's going on here?" asked the young man.

"This woman is about to have a Caesarean birth."

"What's so special about that?"

"There is no anesthetic. She has not been given any painkillers at all. Nothing is controlling the pain except her own mind. She has been hypnotized. She is aware of everything that is going on but she feels no pain."

A surgeon cut through her abdomen with a large scalpel. Blood began to flow from the wound and, minutes later, another member of the surgical team gently pulled out the baby. The umbilical cord was tied and cut, and the baby's cries were deafening when it took its first breath. But the mother, still under hypnosis, was fully awake and in complete control, free of any pain or discomfort.

"This is absolutely amazing!" enthused the young man.

"Hold on, there is more."

The next scene was of a little girl whose skin was covered with red sores.

"This child had a very acute case of eczema. She had previously been given all manner of medicines including steroid creams and ointments and even several courses of antibiotics, but nothing had been able to help. Yet, after six weeks of intensive hypnotherapy, her skin completely cleared."

The film then showed the same child six weeks later with a beautifully smooth and clear complexion.

The woman pressed a button and the film stopped. "I think you are beginning to get the gist of it. You can see the extent to which the mind controls our lives," she said. "The Bible says, 'A man is, as he is in his thoughts.' Your mind controls your body and there is very little, if anything, that it cannot do for you. Things you would think are impossible, such as walking on burning coals, eliminating pain, and healing cancer are easy if you use your mind power. All you need to do is focus your thoughts and get rid of disempowering beliefs."

"What are disempowering beliefs?" asked the young man.

"Well, any belief you have that implies you can't achieve something or that something is impossible is disempowering. Do you think any of those people you saw on the video would have put one foot on the coals if they didn't believe they could walk over it without being burned? Of course not. Healing disease and creating health are all a matter of focusing the power of your mind."

"And you focus your mind with visualization and affirmations?" asked the young man.

"Precisely. I see you're a fast learner," said his teacher. "The power is already there inside you. All you have to do is give it something to focus on, and you can do this with visualizations and affirmations."

"How often do they have to be done?" asked the young man.

"Well, you should spend a minimum of 15 minutes three times a day—morning, noon, and evening, and more often if possible—healing your body with your mind using healing visualizations. And the affirmations should be written down and read out aloud as often as possible. You can use any affirmation that makes you feel healthy, such as: 'I am growing more radiantly healthy every day'; 'I am strong, powerful, and vibrantly healthy'; 'All things are now working together for good in my life'; 'Every day, in every way, I am getting better and better.'

"You can even make up your own affirmation. But whatever statement or statements you choose, you must say it out aloud to yourself every day, as many times as possible and at the very least, morning, noon, and evening. This will soon start to impress on your mind the feeling of Abundant Health."

"I must say I am really excited about what I have learned today. It is wonderful to be able to do something positive to help myself," said the young man. "But tell me something: who is the Chinese man who sent me to you?"

"I have no idea who he is or where he comes from. He never did return to collect the books and to tell you the truth, I didn't expect him to. Somehow, I think he ordered those books for me to read to give me guidance and faith at a time when I needed them most. The only thing I know for certain is that he helped save my life. He showed me one of the most important lessons I have ever learned, even to this day."

"What is that?" asked the young man.

"Simply, that there is very little your mind cannot achieve and the main distinction between those people who recover from illness and those who don't, is their belief in their ability to recover. This is the first law of Abundant Health . . . the foundation of all health and disease lies in the mind!"

The woman then pulled a plaque from the shelf behind her. "This says it all for me," she said. On the plaque was an inscription which read:

> The only ones who conquer are those who believe they can.
>
> *Thomas Emerson*

Later that same evening, the young man read over the notes he had made.

The first secret of Abundant Health—the foundation of all health and disease lies in the mind.

The power of the mind can overcome all pain, heal all disease, and help create Abundant Health.

You can focus the mind on health and healing by:

- Healing visualizations (i.e., spend at least 15 minutes, three times a day, doing healing visualizations)

- Healing affirmations (repeating healing affirmations morning, noon, and night and throughout the day)

The young man felt better about himself and more positive about his health. That day, he had seen wonders and learned about powers that he never dreamed were possible. He took out a small card from his pocket and read aloud the words he had written:

Every day, in every way, I am getting better and better.

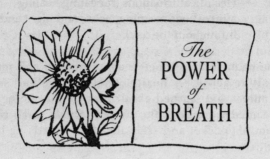

The
POWER
of
BREATH

Two days later the young man sat in a church hall observing a yoga class, waiting to talk to the teacher, a woman by the name of Mrs. Vicki Croft. Hers had been the second name on the old man's list and, like his first teacher, Mrs. Croft had seemed as enthusiastic to meet him as he was to meet her once he had mentioned the little old Chinese man.

After the class, the students thanked their teacher and gradually dispersed, leaving the young man and Mrs. Croft alone. The young man walked over to Mrs. Croft and introduced himself.

"I'm delighted to meet you," Mrs. Croft said with a smile. "So an old Chinese man suggested you come and see me?"

"Yes," replied the young man, "although I'm afraid I don't even know his name."

"I met him only once myself," said Mrs. Croft, "and that was several years ago. But I shall never forget him."

"Why is that?" enquired the young man.

"Because he saved my life!"

The young man was amazed. "Really? He saved your life?"

"Yes. I was suffering from chronic asthma at the time, a problem that had got progressively worse since my childhood. My breathing was labored and, at times, very painful and difficult, although I always managed to control the symptoms with an inhaler. As time passed, it got worse and worse and it seemed that every day I needed more and more puffs from my inhaler. Even walking up the stairs made me wheeze.

"Then one day I had a terrible attack whilst rushing to catch a bus after work. Everyone pushed by me as I gasped for air. I reached for my inhaler but this time it didn't work. It was empty, and at that moment I really thought I was going to die.

"The next thing I remember, a little old Chinese gentleman placed his hand on my back and suddenly the pain was gone. It was quite remarkable. I felt a surge of energy and instantly I was able to breathe. I had never experienced anything like it before, the relief was even better than I would have got from my inhaler. I asked him what he did to me and he said he had released energy that had been blocked in my upper back.

"I didn't really understand what he meant, but I

knew that his presence was a miracle. I never knew his name and I have never met him since, but he saved my life that day.

"He sat with me on a nearby bench whilst I recovered from the shock and it was then that he told me about the laws of Abundant Health and how I could overcome my asthma through them."

"How did you overcome your asthma?" asked the young man.

"Well, I had to change my lifestyle completely, from the foods that I ate to the ways I coped with stress, and the types and amount of exercise I did. There are 10 secrets of Abundant Health and they all are important, but the one which seemed to help me the most was the secret of breath."

"What is that exactly?" asked the young man.

"The difference between life and death lies in our breath. Deep breathing is crucial to our health which is why, if we seek health, we must learn to breathe correctly."

"But what can be 'correct' about breathing?" asked the young man. "We breathe instinctively, don't we?"

"Well, yes, breathing is instinctive and it is a completely natural process, but many people have lost that instinct. When you are sitting down all day, cooped up in air-conditioned offices, and doing little or no exercise, very soon your diaphragm and chest muscles become weak. This makes it virtually impossible for you to breathe correctly."

"Why is it so important to breathe correctly?" asked the young man.

"Breathing is vital to life. Your body can survive weeks without food, and days without water, but starved of oxygen you would not be able to live for more than a few minutes.

"It is something so simple that very few people give it any consideration at all but, nonetheless, it is crucial to health and natural healing. You see, when you breathe you are actually helping to nourish your body because it is oxygen that transports the nutrients you eat around the body. You can eat the best foods in the world and swallow the most expensive and potent vitamin and mineral supplements but they will do you no good whatsoever unless those nutrients can be transported to all of the cells throughout your body, and in order to be transported efficiently, you must breathe well.

"And there are other, equally important benefits of deep breathing," continued Mrs. Croft. "The oxygen that we breathe actually creates energy."

"What do you mean?" asked the young man.

"Well, have you ever seen a log fire?"

"Of course."

"What happens when you blow air on it?"

"The flames grow taller."

"And . . . ?"

"The fire burns brighter?"

"Right again," said Mrs. Croft. "The fire burns brighter! The same thing happens inside your body when your cells burn up calories. Oxygen helps it to burn the calories more efficiently and so creates energy."

"I see, so breathing transports nutrients around our bodies and helps our bodies create energy."

"You're catching on fast. But there's even more to it. Breathing controls the flow of oxygen throughout our bodies and it also controls the flow of lymph in the body."

"What is lymph?" asked the young man.

"Well, lymph is a fluid similar to blood which contains white blood cells to protect your body against bacteria and viruses. It surrounds every one of the 75 trillion cells in your body so, as you can imagine, there is a lot of lymph. In fact, there is over four times more lymph than there is blood. The lymph fluid travels through your body in vessels or tubes very similar to veins and is basically the body's sewage system.

"Here's how it works; blood is pumped from your heart through your arteries and into tiny blood vessels called 'capillaries.' The blood carries the oxygen with the nutrients we have eaten into the capillaries where the oxygen and nutrients are diffused into this fluid around the cells called 'lymph.' Your body's cells know exactly what they need and take the oxygen and nutrients required for their health, and then excrete the toxins. Some toxins find their way back into the capillaries but most dead cells, blood proteins, and other toxic matter are removed by the lymph system."

"I see," said the young man. "But what makes the lymph system work?"

"That's a very good question. The lymph system in your body is activated primarily by two things—exercise and deep breathing. In fact, research has shown that moderate physical exercise coupled with deep breathing exercises can accelerate the rate of lymph drainage by as much as 15 times. Yes, that's 1,500 percent improvement simply by deep breathing and moderate physical exercise!"

The young man was amazed and wrote down notes so as not to forget what he was being told.

"Your body's cells depend upon the lymph to drain excess fluid and toxic wastes," Mrs. Croft explained. "If they were not removed, toxic wastes would accumulate inside your body. Can you imagine what would happen if you did not empty your dustbin regularly at home?"

"It certainly wouldn't smell too good!"

"Precisely. That is because molds and fungus would form, and rats and cockroaches would appear."

The young man nodded.

"Well, when toxic wastes are not removed from the body the same thing happens—bacteria form and parasite organisms and viruses invade. This is one important reason why athletes, for instance, suffer fewer chronic degenerative diseases such as cancer, heart disease, and diabetes than the general population. In fact, according to a recent medical study, nonathletes are seven times more likely to get these diseases than athletes."

The young man scribbled down more notes as Mrs. Croft continued.

"Breathing techniques are also useful in controlling pain. So much so that most pregnant women are taught special breathing exercises to help minimize the pain of childbirth.

"There is also one more very important health benefit in learning to breathe correctly," she said, "and that is its effect on our emotions. Deep breathing relaxes the chest muscles and has a calming effect on the entire nervous system."

"Is this why people are advised to take a deep breath whenever they feel nervous or agitated?" asked the young man.

"Precisely," said the teacher. "I used to be very nervous giving a lecture on yoga but once I took a deep breath I immediately felt calmer and more relaxed. And look at smokers. It is not the cigarette that relaxes them so much as the deep breathing. The only problem being that the toxins from the cigarette congest and destroy the lungs."

"It all makes such good sense," said the young man, "but how can I learn to breathe correctly?"

"A very good question," said the teacher, "and the answer is very simple, you must re-teach your lungs how to breathe. Clinical studies have been carried out in California in which cameras were inserted into people's bodies to record what method of deep breathing exercise had the most positive impact on the lymph and blood circulation. They found that the following exercise was the most effective way of oxygenating your body and stimulating the flow of lymph.

"Try to breathe in the following ratio: inhaling for one count, holding for four counts, and exhaling for two counts. Therefore, if you inhale for four seconds, you should hold your breath for 16 seconds and exhale for eight seconds. Take 10 deep breaths in this ratio—one for inhale, four for hold, and two for exhale. Don't strain yourself. Start by inhaling for three or four seconds and build up slowly. Breathe from your abdomen and imagine your chest is like a vacuum cleaner sucking all of the toxins out of your body."

"I see," said the young man. "But why must I exhale for twice as long as I inhale?"

"Because it is during the time that you exhale that you eliminate toxins via your lymphatic system."

"And why must I hold my breath for four times as long as I inhale?"

"Because that is what fully oxygenates the blood and activates the lymphatic system."

"How often should this exercise be done?" asked the young man.

"Well, it should be done at least three times each day—morning, noon, and night—and gradually your lungs will begin to breathe more deeply throughout the day without you having to think about it. Correct, deep, diaphragmatic breathing will become part of your instinct once again.

"Just try that one simple exercise and within 10 days you will have increased your energy and be feeling a different person."

"I will. Thank you. This really has been very enlightening," said the young man.

"You are very welcome," said Mrs. Croft. "It's always a pleasure to pass on what I have learned. It certainly improved my health beyond my wildest dreams."

That night the young man read over his notes.

The second secret of Abundant Health—the difference between life and death lies in our breath.

Deep breathing:

- is vital to help overcome disease and maintain health

- improves blood and lymph circulation
- relaxes the nervous system
- helps create energy
- relieves mental and emotional stress
- nourishes, cleanses, and relaxes the entire body and calms the mind
- Can be learned by doing the following exercise morning, noon, and night:
  - inhale for as long as is comfortable
  - hold your breath for four times the length of the inhalation
  - exhale for twice as long as the inhalation
  - repeat 10 times

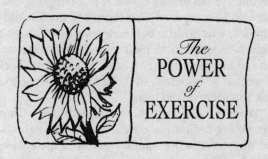

The
POWER
of
EXERCISE

The young man met the third person on his list the following afternoon by the side of the running track in the corner of the city park. She was a lady by the name of Mary O'Donnell, the university track and field team coach. Mary was a fresh-faced woman who arrived dressed in a jade tracksuit, running shoes, and a hair band. They sat together on the front bench in the small grandstand overlooking the running track.

"It was many years ago that I met the old man," Mary said, "but I can remember it so clearly even to this day. It was the same day that I was diagnosed as having MS—multiple sclerosis. As you may know, MS is a disease in which the entire central nervous system breaks down. It is a crippling disease that affects every body function. My doctor told me that there was no cure but there were medications that might help slow down the progress of the disease. As you can imagine, the news came as a terrible shock. It all seemed so hopeless. In the afternoon I came to this park and sat here and wept.

"When I looked up there was an elderly Chinese man sitting beside me on the bench. We got talking and the conversation quickly got onto the subject of natural healing and secrets of health. It was the first time I had ever heard of such things and it certainly gave me a lot to think about. Before the old man left he gave me a list of people who, he said, could help me and he also gave me an article from a health journal that he said I would find interesting.

"I found the article more than interesting. It was incredible. It specifically referred to MS."

"Why was that so incredible?" asked the young man.

"I hadn't told the old man I had MS. I had merely said I had some health problems!

"The article mentioned numerous people who actually recovered from MS. I was very excited because it was the first time I had been given any hope at all that I might be able to get better. I decided that if they could beat it, so could I. Fortunately, in my case, the disease was still in its very early stages and although I was weak, I could still walk."

"How did they recover?" asked the young man.

"Well, it seemed that there were several common factors including diet, mental attitude, and physical exercise.

"I learned the secrets of Abundant Health and immediately put what I had learned into practice. I changed my diet and lifestyle completely. It all paid off, but the thing that brought about the most dramatic improvement in my health was, without a doubt, physical aerobic exercise."

"What do you mean by 'aerobic' exercise?" asked the young man.

"Any exercise that makes your lungs work harder and breathe more rapidly. 'Aerobic' literally means 'to exercise with air.' Brisk walking, running, cycling, and swimming are all good examples. I started to do brisk walking and swimming every day, and although it was difficult at first, because my legs felt like lead, I persevered and gradually my legs got stronger. Within a few months I had improved so much that I was even able to jog in the park.

"I started to jog regularly around the track until I could do as much as eight laps, but it was always at that point that my legs became very tired. A ninth lap was always one lap too many for me, but one day I decided that I had to beat it. If I did nothing else, I was going to run that ninth lap.

"I took it slowly but my legs began to feel heavy just as they always had done as I was completing the eighth lap. I went on a few more paces but the weakness got worse and my legs felt as bad as they had done when the disease had first struck. I really felt as if I couldn't walk another step, let alone run. But suddenly a voice behind me said, 'Keep going, you can do it. Don't give up now.' I turned and who should I see running alongside me? The old Chinese man. He looked at me and smiled, and then said, 'Keep going, you are nearly there!'

"Somehow his words gave me the strength I needed to go on. With the old man running next to me I completed another lap and it was just as well I did, because it was then that the most dramatic change in my health occurred.

"As I began that ninth lap my body broke out into a profuse sweat. It was as if a dam had broken inside me and sweat literally poured out. I suddenly realized that this was the first time I remembered sweating for years and then I was running stronger and faster than ever before. I knew then that it had been a major breakthrough for me. It was perhaps the most important stage in my recovery and since then I have never looked back."

"So what you are saying is that physical exercise played an important part in your recovery?" said the young man as he scribbled some notes.

"Absolutely," said Mary. "Although I had to push myself beyond my limitations before the most dramatic improvement occurred, but for most people the simple act of doing regular light aerobic exercise is often enough."

Just then a middle-aged man walked briskly past them and said, "Morning, Mary."

"Hi Stan, how are you today?"

"Oh, couldn't be better," he replied.

"You wouldn't believe that he had a heart attack last year, would you?" the woman said to the young man.

"Seriously?" said the young man.

"Yes. Regular exercise has helped to save his life as

well. You see, regular aerobic exercise such as running, walking, swimming, and cycling lowers your blood pressure and reduces serum cholesterol in the bloodstream and therefore is of great benefit to the cardiovascular system."

The young man scribbled more notes as she talked.

"You see that lady jogging over there?" Mary pointed to a woman wearing shorts and a sweatshirt. "She had chronic pains in her knees and hips that her doctor had said were arthritis, but it all disappeared within a few weeks when she began doing daily exercise.

"This is because exercise improves the circulation of bodily fluids within the joints, helping to keep them free from arthritic problems—it even helps the bones stay healthy. In fact, lack of exercise actually causes muscle weakness, poor circulation, and calcium loss from the bones which leads to osteoporosis or brittle bones.

"Exercise is so crucial to our health. We simply were not designed to live sedentary lifestyles. Did you know that if you were to bind up your arm for just three days, in that short space of time, the muscles in your arm would already have started to atrophy or waste?"

"Really?"

"Yes, it's like the old saying—if you don't use it, you lose it! Without physical exercise, the whole body weakens. Action brings power. This is the third law of Abundant Health."

The young man was astonished at what he was hearing. He had always known that exercise was important for good health, but he had no idea it was this important. He thought about how little he had exercised in the past few years. No wonder, he thought, he had become so weak.

"Exercise is also important for our mental well-being," continued Mary. "Not many people realize that the less exercise they do, the more prone they become to introversion, anxiety, over-sensitivity, and depression. This is because our emotions are actually influenced by our motion or movement, or lack of it. Clinical studies have shown that exercise helps relieve minor mental disturbances including anxiety and even depression. That's why, when you feel a bit low, getting up and doing some physical activity often helps raise your spirits."

"But why," the young man asked, "should physical exercise affect your emotions?"

"Simple," said Mary. "First, because exercise causes your brain to release morphine-like chemicals called beta-endorphins which produce a feeling of emotional well-being. Many runners experience a mental lift after training and it has become known as 'runners' high.' Secondly, exercise helps our emotional state because our emotions are actually governed by our physiology or the way we hold our bodies. You see, the way we walk, the way we stand or sit, even the way we breathe, all of these movements actually influence our emotional state.

"So you see, regular aerobic exercise is often a vital part in overcoming many physical and mental diseases and is crucial to maintaining Abundant Health," said Mary.

"I see," said the young man. "But what is the best

form of exercise? And how long each day is it best to exercise for?"

"Well, really any exercise you enjoy that causes you to perspire and breathe a little faster. Brisk walking, light jogging, swimming, cycling, and even dancing are all excellent forms of exercise. Start off gently and slowly build up. It is very important to warm up your muscles and joints before doing strenuous exercise otherwise you are likely to 'pull' or 'tear' a muscle or wrench a joint."

"What is the best way to warm up?" asked the young man.

"Well, the easiest way is to try and stretch every muscle and joint for seven seconds at a time, several stretches for each part of your body. All muscles work in pairs and so you should remember that after you stretch one way, you should then stretch the other way."

"I see," said the young man. "Is there anything else I should be aware of?"

"Yes. It is also very important not to overstrain yourself. Build up slowly. Many people make the mistake of trying to do too much exercise too quickly and this often causes injuries from muscle strain."

"I see," said the young man. "And how much exercise is necessary for good health?"

"That's a good question," she answered. "All that is needed is somewhere between 30–60 minutes each day, and within 10 days, I assure you, you will notice a great difference. In fact, the benefits to your health will absolutely astound you as they did me."

"It sounds fantastic," enthused the young man, "I'm going to start exercising today."

"Good luck, and please let me know how you get on," said Mary.

"Of course I will," said the young man. "Thanks for seeing me. I always knew that exercise was important but I never appreciated just how important it is. Oh, by the way, what did the old Chinese man say when you completed the ninth lap?"

"I don't know. When I finished the lap, I turned to thank the old man for his encouragement, but . . . he was no longer there. But of course, now I know he knows," said Mary.

"How?" asked the young man.

"Because every so often I receive a call from someone like you!"

The young man walked away leaving the woman to begin her stretching and warming-up exercises. When the young man reached the park exit, he turned back. The once-crippled woman was jogging around the track in a graceful and seemingly effortless movement, running as if carried by the wind.

The young man felt even more optimistic and confident about improving his own state of health as he checked the notes he had made of his talk with Mary.

The third secret of Abundant Health—action brings power.

Regular physical exercise:

- improves circulation
- strengthens the heart and lungs
- helps overcome many physical and mental

diseases and is essential to maintaining Abundant Health.

Do a form of exercise that you enjoy which:

- makes you perspire
- causes your heart to pump faster
- requires your lungs to work harder.

Always warm your muscles up before strenuous exercise and never strain yourself.
Do at least 30 minutes of physical exercise each day.

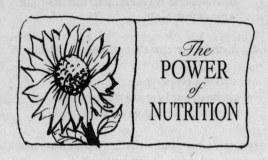

The
POWER
of
NUTRITION

Two days later the young man sat at the corner table of a small but very popular restaurant in the center of town, called *Country Cuisine*. Sitting opposite him was the restaurant proprietor, the fourth person on the young man's list.

Mr. Edward Just was well known and respected throughout the town. Over 80 years old, he clearly loved his work and was always bounding with energy. He still gave cookery classes every week on a Wednesday evening. He was a man with a mission, to teach healthy eating and show how meals could be both delicious and very easy to prepare.

"Your telephone call brought back memories for me," Mr. Just said to the young man. "Wonderful

memories . . . when I was 55 years old, nearly 30 years
ago . . . "

"You are kidding me," the young man interrupted.
"You mean to say you are over 80?"

"Yes, of course."

"My goodness, you don't look a day over 50."

"Thank you," the old man replied with a smile.
"Let me show you something," he said, as he handed
a black-and-white photograph to the young man.

"Who is this?" asked the young man.

"You tell me."

"I don't know. Whoever he is, he looks like he
needs to learn the secrets of Abundant Health."

The photograph showed an immense middle-aged
man, grossly overweight, with a sallow face and dark
shadows under his eyes. You didn't have to be a doctor to realize that this man was unwell.

"It's me," admitted Mr. Just.

"You are joking!" exclaimed the young man.

"No, that really was me. Thirty years ago I was
quite a different person from the man you see before
you. The way I was going I wouldn't have made it
another two years, never mind 30."

"What was wrong with you?" asked the young man.

"'What was right?' would be a better question!"
replied Mr. Just. "I was diabetic for a start."

"But isn't diabetes supposed to be incurable?"
asked the young man.

"That is what people are led to believe, certainly.
But it is not true. Look at me. Many diseases that used
to be thought to be 'incurable' are now being cured.
Not through drugs I might add, but through natural
remedies and changes in lifestyle."

The young man thought about the other people he had seen on the old man's list and how all of them, without exception, had changed his or her lifestyle to overcome their health problem.

The young man's host continued. "I also suffered from high blood pressure, stomach ulcers, and irritable bowels.

"My doctor gave me a collection of different medications and steroids, and at first they seemed to help. But after a few weeks I started getting side effects from the medicines—headaches, nausea, and then skin rashes. I was continuously tired and my health got steadily worse until one day a chance meeting with an old man changed my life."

"An old Chinese man, I suppose?" interrupted the young man.

"Yes, of course," smiled Mr. Just.

"What happened?"

"It was most strange. In those days, my job was very stressful and I rarely even had time to leave the office for lunch. Yet, one day I felt so terrible that I decided to go out for lunch to a small café which was just across the road from my office. I sat in the corner eating a cheeseburger and chips when an old Chinese gentleman asked if he could join me.

"The old man sat down and ate a large salad and baked potato. We exchanged pleasantries and then, quite out of the blue, he looked me straight in the eye and said that the food I was eating was killing me. I made a joke of it but he persisted and then he said something that really shocked me . . . He said that the food I was eating was aggravating my stomach ulcers!"

"Why did that shock you?" asked the young man.

"Because I hadn't mentioned my ulcers to him. I asked him how he knew I had stomach ulcers and he told me he could see it in my eyes."

"Really?" enquired the young man.

"Yes. It sounds incredible, I know, but true nonetheless. I was intrigued by what the Chinese man had said and I asked him what else he 'saw.' Would you believe he told me that I had dangerously high levels of cholesterol and a weak pancreas.

"So I asked him, what should I be eating, if the food I was eating was killing me? It was then that he told me about the secrets of Abundant Health. He patiently explained that health can only be created through healthy living which involved following the Laws of Nature that produce health in abundance. There are 10 laws of Abundant Health which, if followed, actually produce abundant health; but if they are broken, they will just as surely produce disease. They are all important but the one with which I can help you most, is the Law of Abundant Nutrition—you are what you eat, when you eat, and how you eat.

"After I met the Chinese man that day, I went to see several people about my health. The first thing I changed was my diet, and I made some major changes in what, when, and how I ate. Would you believe that within six weeks my cholesterol levels were back to normal, my ulcers had gone, and I hadn't had one attack of heartburn! And the most incredible thing of all . . . my diabetes was cured!"

"'That's unbelievable!" said the young man.

"It is, isn't it?" said Mr. Just. "But it's true. I have

since read of clinical studies in which 75 percent of adult diabetic patients who were put on a low-fat, high-fiber diet were completely cured within eight weeks!"

"I knew then that there is something very powerful in the Law of Abundant Nutrition and I decided to learn about the science of nutrition in detail. I learned that healthy eating can be summarized into six simple rules which, without doubt, can help anybody overcome many diseases and maintain abundant health."

The young man was listening more intently now and busily writing down notes as Mr. Just spoke.

"The first rule of healthy eating is to choose wholesome, fresh, unrefined foods. Good nutrition is like building a house. Your house will only be as sound as the materials with which it is built, you agree?"

The young man nodded, but was unsure what the difference was between "unrefined" and "refined" foods.

"Refined foods," explained Mr. Just, "are those foods that have had all the goodness taken out of them such as white bread, white sugar, and even packaged breakfast cereals. Most of the vitamins, minerals, and other nutrients are extracted or destroyed in the process and these foods are generally just full of sugar and starch."

"But I eat white bread and packaged breakfast cereal and it says on the wrappers that they are 'enriched with added vitamins,'" protested the young man.

"That's just misleading advertising. What the manufacturers actually do is take 100 nutrients out of the food and then put five artificial vitamins back. I don't know about you, but I'd hardly call that 'enriched'!"

"But what is so harmful about sugar and starch anyway?" persisted the young man. "I thought they gave you energy."

"Well, it's true that sugars and starches are needed to produce energy but so are many other nutrients including calcium, zinc, iron, and many other minerals and vitamins. Most of these nutrients are missing from refined foods and so your body has to take them from its own bones and tissues. Consequently, the body's stores of many essential minerals and vitamins become depleted, the 'refined' foods actually rob your body of vital resources."

"So what are all the 'unrefined' foods we should eat?"

"Fresh fruits and vegetables; whole grains such as brown rice, wholemeal bread, barley, oats, millet, and rye. Then there are pulses and beans, nuts, and seeds. These are the whole foods that form the basis of a healthy diet. They contain proteins, carbohydrates, vitamins, minerals, and essential fatty acids all in the proportion Nature intended for you.

"Of course, where possible, organically grown foods are best."

"What are 'organically grown foods'?" asked the curious young man.

"Foods which are grown without the use of chemical fertilizers, pesticides, or any chemical treatments. All of the chemicals used in commercial agricultural methods are potentially toxic. Organic foods—which are grown naturally—have no such chemical residues in them and they have much higher amounts of nutrients.

"The second rule of healthy eating is that you cannot have good nutrition without good digestion. Remember, we are not just what we eat, we are when and how we eat!"

"I'm not sure what you mean," said the young man.

"It's no good eating wholesome foods if you cannot digest them, and the only way to ensure good digestion is to eat at the right times and in the proper manner. For instance, it is difficult to digest food properly if you don't chew each mouthful thoroughly. Similarly, your body cannot digest food well when you are angry or tired or rushing whilst eating.

"Many people 'grab' a meal. They eat it in a hurry in between jobs and then wonder why they suffer indigestion. Eating should be relaxed and the food enjoyed. When you savor food, your mouth produces more saliva which is needed to digest carbohydrates and the stomach can more easily produce hydrochloride acid to digest protein. But perhaps the greatest obstacle to healthy digestion is the time at which we eat."

"What has the time at which we eat got to do with digestion?" asked the young man.

"The whole of Nature works according to set and very precise times," explained Mr. Just. "From the setting of the sun to the flowering of a tulip, everything has its time and the human body is no exception. It has its own built-in clock, more precise and finely tuned than we could possibly imagine. The time at which we eat is very important in determining how well food will be digested.

"For instance, your body's metabolic rate—the rate at which your body converts food into energy—is much slower in the evening than in the morning. This means that calories are burned much less efficiently. This is why, if you eat the bulk of your food in the evening, you tend to put on more weight than if you were to eat the bulk of your food in the morning.

"And on top of that, if you eat late at night you tend not to get good quality sleep. More likely than not, you will wake up tired in the morning."

"Why is that?" asked the young man.

"When we eat in the evening the digestive system has to work throughout the night; the brain gets no rest because it has to send messages to the stomach and intestines to produce the necessary digestive enzymes and juices."

"I see," said the young man. "Are there any other times when it is not good to eat?"

"Yes, when you are very tired or very stressed because when you are in these states the digestive system does not function very well and consequently foods are not well digested."

The young man busily scribbled notes as Mr. Just continued.

"The third rule for healthy eating is never overeat.

"Remember, when you eat—less is more. It is far easier for you to eat small amounts of food than large amounts. A healthy stomach is only the size of your fist. When we overeat, the stomach expands under the strain and this impedes the digestive process much like putting too much coal into a boiler stifles the heat. More importantly, excess calories create additional fat which burdens the heart as well as putting additional strain on the joints. It is for this reason that people who eat less live longer. There is an old saying, 'Eat until your stomach is half full, drink until your thirst is half quenched, and you will be sure to live a full life.'"

"The fourth rule of healthy eating is that 70 percent of the diet should be made up of water-rich foods— fresh fruits, vegetables, and sprouted grains and pulses. The other 30 per cent should be made up of the starches, proteins, and fats. This may seem strange, bearing in mind that the average person in the western world eats a small proportion of water-rich foods and a high proportion of starches and proteins—lots of meat, lots of bread and potatoes and few vegetables. But the average person in the western world is ill. One in three gets cancer, one in two dies of heart-related disease. And think about it for a moment; the earth is 70 percent water, the human body is 70 percent water. Doesn't it make sense to eat foods in the same ratio?"

"Why can't we just drink more water?" asked the young man.

"That's a good point," said Mr. Just. "In the first place most of the water people drink isn't very pure. Chances are it contains chlorine, fluoride, soft metals, and other toxic substances. But in any event, you can't cleanse your system by drowning it. Just as we should eat only when we are hungry, we should drink only when we are thirsty. A diet centered around water-rich foods is cleansing and nourishing.

If we do not have enough fluid, the blood in our bodies becomes too thick and poisonous wastes cannot be eliminated efficiently. Our diets should contain foods which assist the body in building and cleansing itself."

The young man thought for a moment about how many water-rich foods he usually ate and the answer horrified him—very, very few. He ate mostly meats, potatoes, bread and butter, with the odd cooked vegetable.

"The fifth rule of healthy eating," continued Mr. Just, "is very important—avoid the five 'cell destroyers.'"

"What are the cell destroyers?" asked the young man.

"Cell destroyers are those foods which are particularly harmful to your health because they destroy your body's cells. These are foods that should be avoided as much as possible. The less you have of them, the better off you'll be, and I'll explain why.

"The first cell destroyer is refined sugar. Sugar is a deadly food. Apart from rotting your teeth, it is a refined food and therefore depletes your body of its vital resources. But it also destroys your immune system. Did you know that just six teaspoons of sugar will reduce the number of your white blood cells—the cells which fight germs and bacteria—by 25 percent? And the more sugar you eat, the more cells are destroyed.

"Remember that sugar is often disguised in many other foods such as sweets, chocolates, cold drinks, cakes and biscuits, and even in tinned fruit and vegetables.

"The second cell destroyer is flesh foods—meat, poultry, and fish. Let's consider meat and poultry first; research studies have shown time and time again that the one single major factor in most chronic, degenerative diseases is the consumption of meat. For a start, most meat today comes from factory-farmed animals. This means that the animals are kept in 'factory' conditions—caged in box-tight compartments, never to graze open pastures, never even to know sunlight. Pumped with antibiotics to control the spread of disease in such terrible conditions and fed with hormones and growth promoters, it is no surprise that the meat becomes polluted with a cocktail of poisons."

"But what about vegetables and fruits?" asked the young man. "Aren't they also sprayed with dangerous chemicals?"

Mr. Just smiled. "Very true," he said, "very true. But these are very minuscule when compared to the pollutants in meat. One professor in Norway compared a commercially grown cabbage to a chicken and found that the chicken had over 10 million more toxins.

"Organic fruits and vegetables are grown without chemicals and are of course far better for you. They are more nutritious and they do not contain health-destroying toxins. But even those that are chemically grown are far, far less toxic than meat."

"But what about 'organic' meat?" persisted the young man.

"Well, there is no doubt that it is better than the meat of factory-farmed animals, but it is still extremely damaging to your health. Meat is simply not a healthy food.

"You see, meat and poultry are very high in saturated fats—these are fats which cause the red blood cells to stick together and clog up the arteries. It is therefore not surprising that half of the population die from heart-related diseases and the vast majority of them are caused by the excess fat and cholesterol found in meat, dairy foods, and chocolate."

"But I always thought meat was good for health," said the young man. "Don't we need meat for energy?"

"Not at all, in fact the reverse is true. The first thing the body burns for energy is carbohydrates. Meat contains very little carbohydrate but a lot of fat and protein, and excess protein in the body leads to excess nitrogen and excess nitrogen creates fatigue."

"But, I heard you need plenty of meat for strong bones," said the young man.

"Again, quite the reverse is true. People who eat meat have the weakest bones because meat contains an awful lot of uric acid. Uric acid is what gives meat its taste, but it is also highly toxic. You see, your body can only eliminate about eight grains of uric acid each day, yet a quarter-pound beefburger contains up to sixteen grains. This excess irritates the tendons and joints, creating arthritis, and it also leeches calcium from your bones."

"But what about iron?" asked the young man. "Where can you get enough iron if you don't eat meat?"

"You get plenty of iron in green leafy vegetables and cereals and pulses. In fact, calorie for calorie, lentils, spinach, broccoli, and even dried apricots contain more iron than beef steak. One cup of brown rice has more iron than a quarter-pound hamburger. It is a fallacy that vegetarians suffer from anemia more than meat eaters. And recent medical studies have actually revealed that excess iron is linked to heart disease."

"But why is fish so bad?" asked the young man. "I thought fish was good for you."

"Fish may not be as bad for you as meat, but it is certainly not a healthy food. Many seas are so polluted that government surveys have found nearly half of all fish have cancerous growths. And farmed fish, like farmed animals, are fed a plethora of antibiotics to control disease levels, hormones to promote rapid growth, and chemical colorants to turn the flesh pink.

"Fish has been promoted as a health food because it has Omega-3 essential fatty acids which are thought to help people suffering from heart disease and arthritis. However, the fat cells in fish are heavily polluted and not only do some vegetable oils have higher amounts of Omega-3 essential fatty acids than fish, but medical studies have also shown them to be more effective.

"The flesh of other creatures, be it meat or fish, is simply not a natural food for humans. Humans are herbivorous by nature; herbivores have jaws that move laterally and vertically, with teeth suitable for grinding, while carnivores' jaws only move up and down, their teeth rip and tear, not grind. Herbivores have typically over 22 feet of intestines but carnivores have only about three feet so that the flesh is expelled before it has time to putrefy. Most anthropologists agree that man was originally a fruit-picking primate.

"All of the nutrients we need are provided in a meatless diet. In my day, vegetarians were considered cranks but this was an image created by the media. Who do you think those cranks were? They were the great thinkers and philosophers throughout history from Socrates, Pythagoras, and Plato in ancient Greece, to the more modern times including Leonardo da Vinci, Henry David Thoreau, Albert Einstein, Isaac Newton, Benjamin Franklin, George Bernard Shaw, Leo Tolstoy, H. G. Wells, Mark Twain, Voltaire, and Gandhi. Hardly a list of cranks! And don't forget most of them lived very long, healthy lives too."

The young man busily wrote notes as Mr. Just continued.

"The third cell destroyer is dairy food—all milk, cheese, cream, and butter. Human beings are the only creatures on earth to drink another creature's milk and the only creatures to drink milk beyond infancy."

"But what is so bad about dairy foods?" asked the young man, who by now was seriously worried that there would be nothing left to eat that was actually good for you other than lettuce leaves and carrots.

"Dairy food is fine for calves but not for humans. Twenty percent of the population do not produce lactase which is needed to digest lactose, the sugar in milk. And it has been estimated that four out of five people are allergic to the principal protein in dairy foods, called 'casein.'

"Dairy foods are one of the most destructive foods you can eat. They create a tremendous amount of mucus in your body which affects digestion because the mucus lines the stomach and intestines and hardens, forming a barrier through which nutrients cannot pass. Mucus also accumulates in the lungs and causes many respiratory disorders including bronchitis and asthma.

"Dairy foods contain very high amounts of fat and that, as I mentioned, causes many heart-related diseases."

"But don't we need dairy food for calcium?" asked the young man.

"Not at all," explained Mr. Just. "In fact, studies have shown that the people who have the highest intake of dairy food also have the lowest levels of calcium. For example, the people of Norway are amongst the highest consumers of dairy food in the world but they also have one of the highest rates of osteoporosis (or brittle bones) in the world. On the other hand, the Bantu people in Africa consume less than one quarter the calcium intake of western societies yet they suffer no diseases related to calcium deficiency, rarely even breaking a bone or losing a tooth. The reason? Their lower-protein diet does not throw calcium out of the body in the way the high-protein diet in western countries does.

"The calcium in dairy foods simply cannot be absorbed well and often becomes deposited around the joints, causing arthritis, and on the artery walls, causing hardening of the arteries. And think about it; a cow eats mainly grass, which has virtually no calcium, yet produces large quantities of calcium in her milk. Likewise, humans get all the calcium they need from green leafy vegetables and cereals. For example, a cup of chopped broccoli contains far more calcium than a cup of milk.

"The fourth cell destroyer is table salt or sodium chloride."

"What's wrong with table salt? I thought your body needs sodium," said the young man.

"Your body does need sodium; it helps maintain a healthy fluid balance, assists muscle power, helps the proper functioning of your nervous system, and maintains the correct balance of acids in your blood and urine. But we get plenty of sodium in fruits and vegetables such as tomatoes, celery, spinach, kale, carrots, and even strawberries. All the sodium our bodies need can be obtained in the vegetables and whole foods we eat. Excess sodium can be very harmful.

"Most people eat far too much sodium in the form of table salt. For instance, your body needs approximately 3000 milligrams of sodium every day, depending upon your lifestyle—you can lose a lot in perspiration. One teaspoon of table salt has about 2,000 milligrams! Consequently, many people can have four or five times too much sodium if they use table salt or eat a lot of canned foods and processed foods because they also contain very large quantities of salt.

"Table salt is an inorganic sodium which has been bleached and refined. It irritates the stomach and hinders the digestion of other foods. If you do have any salt for seasoning, it is much better to use sea salt because it is unrefined, unbleached, and contains essential minerals and trace elements which your body needs. However, remember excess sodium can cause water retention which restricts the amount of oxygen reaching the cells in your body, and can even lead to high blood pressure. In fact, most heart disease patients and many people with liver and kidney problems are put on low-sodium diets by their doctors. Doesn't it make sense to shut the stable door before the horse bolts?

"The fifth cell destroyer is tea, coffee, and alcohol."

"I knew, of course, excess alcohol was not good for your health because it harms the kidneys and liver, but what is wrong with tea and coffee?" asked the young man.

"Tea and coffee, like alcohol, are stimulants that harm the body. For instance, both tea and coffee contain caffeine which is a potent drug. Two cups of tea or coffee contain a pharmaceutical dose of caffeine which is enough to stimulate the brain and raise our blood sugar level. You may feel more alert at first, but it quickly wears off. Your blood sugar level will then fall below the point where it first started leaving you feeling more tired than before.

"And have you noticed when you drink several cups of tea or coffee, you become more nervous and your heart pumps faster? Sometimes it can actually cause your hands to tremble."

The young man nodded. It was true, he remembered only a few weeks earlier when one night his hands had been shaking slightly after he had drunk four mugs of coffee in succession.

Mr. Just continued: "And caffeine does more damage than just stimulating your nervous system and raising sugar levels in your blood—it increases your blood pressure, causes a rise in cholesterol, irritates the stomach, burns up the body's stores of vitamin B, and the high oxalic acid content in tea and coffee can even damage your kidneys. One researcher in food allergies claimed that caffeine is one of the main foods causing allergic reactions including insomnia, headaches, nervousness, irritability, and skin complaints.

"Tea has an added drug called 'tannin' which can interfere with the body's absorption of iron and lead to anemia.

"Whilst in small quantities, tea and coffee are harmless, when they are drunk in excess, i.e., more than two cups per day, they can be very harmful indeed."

The young man thought carefully about the five rules of healthy eating and was painfully aware that he had not lived by any of them. No wonder he was so ill. But he felt depressed about the whole subject of nutrition.

"I understand what you say," he said to Mr. Just, "but what is there left that I can eat? It seems a bit dreary to live off cabbage leaves and salad."

"Oh, it's not like that at all. Natural wholesome food does not have to be tasteless. It can be the most delicious food you could possibly imagine. Come, let me show you."

They walked to the center of the room where there was a huge colorful selection of different dishes. On one table was a choice of two soups—cream of broccoli and leek and potato—alongside them were displayed five different freshly baked breads. The young man recognized the rye, granary, and whole wheat, but he had never heard of the millet bread or black bread. Further on there were a variety of beautifully presented dishes. The young man could almost taste the aroma of the freshly cooked herbs. He read the name beside each dish: cooked whole-grain rice with sesame seeds, millet rissoles, sweet potatoes stuffed with zuccini and chestnut, sweet and sour mixed vegetables, Hungarian goulash, as well as a vast selection of raw vegetables and salad stuffs.

On yet another table were bowls of dried fruit, granola, and freshly-sliced fruits. There was even a variety of non-dairy "creams"—almond and strawberry, raspberry and hazelnut, and one that looked and tasted like chocolate made from carob beans.

"I've never seen such a vast selection of food for lunch," said the young man.

"Thank you. We try very hard to please everybody's palate," said his host.

After filling his tray with soup, millet bread, and rice and goulash, the young man made his way back to his chair.

"How do you like it?" asked the old man as the young man took his second mouthful.

"Absolutely delicious. It's really tasty," enthused the young man.

"And it's all very healthy and extremely nutritious," Mr. Just assured him.

The two men ate lunch together and the young man relished every mouthful. It was one of the most delicious meals he had eaten for a long time, and certainly a far cry from his usual burger and chips. He resolved to take more care about the food he ate and to give his body only the best wholesome foods.

After lunch, the young man summarized his notes of the meeting:

The fourth secret of Abundant Health—the power of Abundant Nutrition.

There is no Abundant Health without Abundant Nutrition: you are what you eat, when you eat, and how you eat.

The five rules of Abundant Nutrition:

- Good nutrition is like building a house. Choose wholesome fresh, unrefined, and organic foods.
- Good nutrition requires good digestion. Therefore, chew food well, eat while relaxed, and don't eat late at night or between meals.
- Less is more! Don't overeat.
- Seventy percent of the food we eat should be water-rich foods.
- Avoid as much as possible the cell destroyers—sugar, meat, fish, dairy food, table salt, tea, coffee, and alcohol.

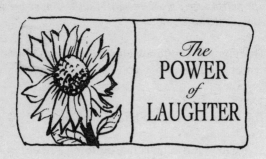

The
POWER
of
LAUGHTER

The next person on the young man's list was a young journalist by the name of Neil Collins. He had a warm face with smiling eyes and exuded a familiar glow and zest for life that the young man had noticed in the other people he had so far met.

"That old Chinese man is someone special, isn't he?" Mr. Collins said to the young man. "Do you know that he showed me a miraculous medicine that saved my life."

"Miraculous medicine?" repeated the young man. "But the old man told me that tablets rarely cure disease!"

"Oh, this medicine doesn't come in a bottle. In fact, this is a medicine that very few doctors prescribe and you certainly won't find it in any pharmacy."

The young man was intrigued. What on earth was the journalist talking about?

Mr. Collins continued: "Yet it is a medicine that has been spoken of for over 3,000 years and, in recent times, it has been proven not only to be important in helping cure many diseases but it has also been shown to be very important in helping to maintain health. It is a simple medicine, available to anybody, anywhere and anytime . . . "

"But what is this medicine?" urged the young man.

"Laughter!" he answered and burst out laughing at the sight of the young man's incredulous expression.

The young man sat in disbelief. "You're joking," he said.

"Not at all," said Mr. Collins. "Let me tell you my story. Ten years ago I was crippled and laid up in a hospital bed suffering from an arthritic disease called Ankylosing Spondylitis. It is a degenerative condition affecting the tissues around the spine and causes severe pain. My prognosis was not good. I was told that less than 1 in 500 people recovers from this disease.

"My condition went from bad to worse. The pain killers were becoming less and less effective and the pain was virtually constant, day and night. I didn't know how much more I could take. I became desperate and was really afraid I might die. Then one day a miracle happened.

"A new doctor came into my room and asked how I was. I told him how bad I was feeling and he said that I needed something better to help relieve the pain. He said he had to meet someone but would return a little while later. In the meantime he suggested I watch a little TV to help take my mind off things. He turned on the television and one of my favorite programs was on, a show called *Cheers*. Have you ever seen *Cheers*?" he asked the young man.

"Yes, it's one of my favorites, too."

"Well, the episode that night was hilarious. It must have been one of the funniest I had ever seen and I just laughed and laughed. At the end of the show, the doctor returned and asked again how I was feeling. It was only then that I noticed ... I had no pain! It was unbelievable. Remember, this was the first time I had been free from pain since my illness had begun."

The doctor was not surprised. He said that laughter was one of the best medicines he knew. We chatted for a while about my health and he gave me the names of some of his colleagues who, he said, would be able to help me once I got out of hospital.

"But several hours later the pain started to return. I was about to get depressed again but all of a sudden it occurred to me."

"What?" asked the young man eager to find out.

"All I needed to do was find something that made me laugh. I arranged for a video recorder to be brought into my room and I watched past episodes of *Cheers* that I had recorded. And just as I had hoped, it worked. The pain subsided again, and again and again. The laughter was actually alleviating my pain. So much so, in fact, that after a few days I decided to discharge myself from hospital because the food was lousy, the air was stuffy, and I felt I would be better off out in the country somewhere with fresh air, pure water, and fresh food. So, I moved into a quiet hotel and watched lots of my favorite funny videos—films and television programs that made me laugh.

"Of course, along with plenty of laughter, I also made sure I had a nutritious diet and plenty of fresh air, and I gradually exercised more and more. There are many things necessary to create a healthy life, many laws in Nature which need to be respected, and I learned them from the people on the doctor's list. But the one thing that stood out most for me in my recovery was simple laughter.

"After four months, the pain had completely gone and the subsequent hospital tests showed that I was completely cured. No trace of anything anywhere. I had overcome a disease that less than 1 in 500 people recovers from using conventional medicine, and yet I had no tablets and no medicines except for a good supply of laughter."

"That's amazing," said the young man, "but why do you think laughter helped you so much?"

"That's an interesting question and one that I asked myself at the time. I did some research and found some incredible studies that showed why laughter is so beneficial to our health. You see, laughter has a wonderful effect on our bodies. For instance, it causes the brain to release hormone-like chemicals known as 'endorphins' which are a natural pain killer and also help boost our immune system.

"Laughter also increases our respiratory activity, exercising the heart and lungs, which enables us to take in more oxygen, and obtaining sufficient oxygen is absolutely essential to our health."

"Yes, I learned how important breathing is to our health from a yoga teacher a few weeks ago," interrupted the young man.

"Well, laughter is one of the most enjoyable and effective ways of improving your lung capacity, and a good belly laugh also stimulates the bowels and massages the organs and tissues in the abdomen. This, in effect, means that the blood supply to all of your vital organs is improved every time you laugh."

"Laughing also helps our mental health too. Several studies have shown that people concentrate better after they have laughed, and laughter even reduces the effects of stress. For instance, did you know that the body's stress hormones—adrenaline and cortisol—are lowered when we laugh?

"Look at this," said the journalist as he reached for a book on his shelf. It was the Bible and he flicked through the pages until he found what he was looking for. "Here it is. Read this. Proverbs 17:22," and he handed it to the young man.

The passage read:

A merry heart doeth good like a medicine.

"Those words were written over 3,000 years ago. The medical profession still ignores them, but believe you me, never were truer words written. Laughter is a medicine that really will help you overcome any disease and it will also help you stay healthy."

It was then that the young man realized how little he had laughed in the past months. Caught up in the stresses and strains of everyday living, he had become tense and serious.

"It's not easy to laugh when life is so stressful."

"Yes, you're absolutely right," said Mr. Collins. "But it is at stressful times that we most need to laugh. All we need to do in a stressful situation is to look for something funny and ask ourselves, 'What's funny about this situation?' or 'What could be funny about this situation?' What you notice in life depends on what you are looking for. If you look for magic, you will lead a magical life; if you look for disasters, you will have a disaster-filled life; but if you look for laughter, you will live a joyous and healthy life.

"And, let me ask you this; haven't you had experiences that seemed upsetting when they happened, but months or years later you laughed about them?"

The young man nodded. He was reminded of an incident years back when, one evening when he was trying to impress a girlfriend, a waiter had tripped and spilled a tray of desserts all over him. He was furious and terribly embarrassed at the time but weeks later he was laughing with friends about it.

"Why wait to laugh about experiences?" continued Mr. Collins. "Why not see the funny side of life as it happens? Life is a drama, but you can make it a tragedy or a comedy . . . it's all up to you, do you see?"

The young man was very excited at this revelation and he was determined to make a change.

"I have got to tell you," he said to Mr. Collins, "that all of this sounds absolutely fantastic and it all makes complete sense. From now on, I will take myself less seriously and I will try to ensure that I get a good dose of laughter every day." He closed his notepad.

"One more thing," he asked, "the doctor who visited you that day, he was the elderly Chinese man, wasn't he?"

"Of course, who else?" replied the journalist. "And I'll tell you something: I knew that a miracle had happened when I went back to see my doctor at the hospital after I had recovered. He told me that he had never witnessed such a profound recovery before in a patient with my condition. I told him it was all thanks to his colleague, the elderly Chinese doctor. He had no idea who I was talking about—there were no Chinese doctors working in the hospital!

"I have no idea myself who the old man is or where he comes from, but I do know he is no ordinary man."

The young man had, of course, suspected that from the outset but the stories of the people he had met confirmed his suspicions. The path to Abundant Health was opening up before him and was leading him to simple truths about healthy living.

"Say, before you go," said the journalist, "have you heard the one about a man who goes into a bar with a crocodile . . . ?"

Outside his office, Mr. Collins's secretary heard the sound of two men taking their favorite medicine . . . laughter.

Later that day the young man read over his notes from his meeting.

The fifth secret of Abundant Health—laughter is a timeless healer.

Laughter is an effective medicine which helps alleviate pain and heal many diseases.

Laughter improves your breathing, exercises your heart and lungs, helps bowel movement, and massages all of the organs in your abdomen.

Laughter boosts your immune system.

Laughter improves concentration and relieves mental stress.

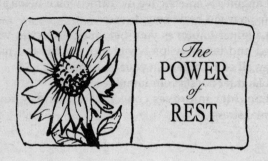

The
POWER
of
REST

It was not until the following week that the young man was able to meet the next person on the old man's list. During that time he had followed the advice he had been given and he was amazed at how much better he had already begun to feel. His family and friends noticed the change as well. If he had any doubts about the secrets of abundant health before, there were none now. He could not remember the last time he had felt so well.

Richard Shaw was a "Stress Management Consultant" and quite different from other successful businessmen the young man had encountered before. He had a healthy, glowing face with sparkling eyes and a reassuring, calm, and relaxed manner.

"So you want to learn about the secrets of Abundant Health?" Mr. Shaw asked the young man. "I first discovered them 15 years ago. My life was quite different then, I can tell you. I was a very successful stockbroker earning very good money but, at the same time, I was very poor."

"What do you mean?" asked the young man.

"I was in poor health and without your health, what good is money or material possessions? I worked hard, sometimes 16 hours a day, under intense stress. I was dealing with vast sums of money, literally millions of pounds every day. One wrong decision could make or lose hundreds of thousands, if not millions, of pounds."

"That is some pressure!" agreed the young man.

"It certainly is, believe me. But the pressure soon began to take its toll. I found it more and more difficult to relax and in the end I resorted to drinking alcohol to calm myself down at the end of each day. Sometimes I was so tense that I even took tranquillizers. Over the years I managed to turn myself into a physical and nervous wreck. I suffered with high blood pressure, stomach ulcers, and the most terrible migraine headaches. Although I was earning plenty of money, as far as my health was concerned I was a bankrupt living on borrowed time."

"So what brought about the change?" asked the young man.

"A train journey," replied Mr. Shaw.

The young man looked surprised. "What do you mean?" he said.

"One day I was traveling home on a train which was suddenly delayed between stations. It was very crowded and, the longer we were delayed, the more tense and agitated I became. My chest began to tighten and I started struggling to catch my breath. I didn't know it then but I was actually having a heart attack.

"The next thing I remember was lying down looking into the face of an elderly Chinese man who was kneeling beside me. He examined my eyes and told me I had had a mild heart attack and that I was suffering from nervous exhaustion.

"He took me to the local hospital for a thorough examination and on the way he talked to me about the effect my lifestyle was having on my health. It was then that I first learned about the secrets of Abundant Health. I had no idea that simple things like the food we eat or the exercise we do were so important to the state of our health. The old Chinese man gave me a list of people who would teach me the secrets of Abundant Health and I soon found out that my lifestyle had been more conducive to disease than health. But the one thing which I had completely neglected throughout my working life was the sixth law of Abundant Health—the power of rest and relaxation."

"What is that?" enquired the young man.

"Simply this; rest rejuvenates your mind, body, and spirit. You can never attain Abundant Health without resting the body and mind. It's so simple when you think about it, yet it is something we all tend to ignore.

"Every living thing in the world requires rest—people, animals, even the land—it is part of Nature's design. All of the plant and animal kingdom rest at the appropriate time. The Bible mentions that even God rested on the seventh day after he created the world, yet we human beings so often think we can do without it. We rush madly through life at a frantic pace without taking the time to slow down, let alone stop even for a moment. We have no time to watch the glowing sunset on a summer's evening, no time to smell the sweet scent of cherry blossom in spring, and no time to listen to the sound of birds singing. Have you noticed that, in an age where we have so many time-saving devices—telephones, faxes, washing machines, dryers, vacuum cleaners, computers, cars, aeroplanes—people still have no time? It seems that people rush around more than ever.

"The pressures of one day are usually carried into the next and the next . . . and the next. This is why so many people are tired through the day, and suffer chronic fatigue and chronic illnesses.

"I was like so many other people—highly stressed and continuously exhausted. Fortunately for me it was not too late to make amends. I learned to relax and rest properly. As a result, my health changed dramatically. All of my past symptoms disappeared and my blood pressure returned to normal within a few weeks. It was incredible."

"Really?" said the young man, "Simply getting more rest was that important to your recovery?"

"Absolutely," said Mr. Shaw. "Adequate physical and mental rest are essential for our well-being. Scientific research has proven that physical and mental relaxation reduce the amount of oxygen your body requires by as much as 50 percent and the workload of your heart by as much as 30 percent, and lower high blood pressure. Deep relaxation also reduces the amount of lactate in your blood which is a chemical associated with anxiety, neurosis, and high blood pressure. Studies have shown that brain wave patterns become more synchronized, alertness and reaction time are increased, and both short-term and long-term memory are improved after we rest.

"People experience better sleep, fewer headaches, greater physical energy, and better general health. Not to mention the fact that being rested can help improve family and social relationships due to less irritability. There is no doubt that rest and relaxation are vital for your health and well-being."

"This is very interesting but how can you ensure that you are relaxed or that you get enough rest?" asked the young man. "When you're under stress it is so difficult to relax, and you said yourself that you used to resort to alcohol and tranquillizers."

"A very good question that deserves my best answer," said Mr. Shaw. "The first thing to do is learn to rest your mind. Every day we need to take time to stop and contemplate, meditate and relax. Most people cannot work efficiently for more than one hour at a time without a break. Concentration starts to flag and so it is counter-productive to work for long periods of time without a break. Regular short breaks are desperately needed in office life. Employers would find their employees more efficient, making fewer mistakes, and becoming more creative and productive if they allowed them to take regular short breaks. Taking a break for just 10 minutes or so is time very well spent, not only for your health but also for your work. It is all that is needed to rest weary bones and a troubled mind. It's sort of like a mental holiday which calms your nervous system and leaves you feeling re-energized and wonderfully refreshed."

"Don't we do that when we sleep?"

"Not necessarily. It is true that we all need sleep, but have you ever woken up in the morning after a long night's sleep feeling just as tired as when you went to bed?"

The young man nodded. "Yes, quite often actually," he said.

"Then do you think you have been well rested?"

"I suppose not." It suddenly occurred to the young man that although he slept a great deal, he always awoke tired and never felt truly rested.

"Just because you get a lot of sleep does not mean that you get sufficient rest. Sleep is very important; most people need between six and eight hours' sleep a night, but proper rest requires a peaceful or restful attitude otherwise your mind will continue to bother you whilst you are asleep. Most people worry about very small and often very trivial things and this saps our energy and robs us of our rest."

"I am a terrible worrier," said the young man, "always have been."

"Ah, but just because you always have been doesn't necessarily mean that you always will be. The past does not equal the future. It is only when you do the things you have always done, that you get what you have always got! You can change, believe me. There is a simple two-step formula to stop worrying and develop a peaceful attitude.

"What is it?" asked the young man.

"Very simple. Step one is: *Don't worry about the*

small things in life. And step two is: *Remember most things in life are small.*

"We need to take life a little less seriously, and whenever we get uptight and frustrated we should just ask ourselves this question: 'In 10 years from now, will anybody care?' If they won't, it is almost certainly a small thing and therefore does not warrant wasting time worrying over.

"To rest our mind and body we must also learn to take only one day at a time. Jesus said, 'Give us *this* day our daily bread.'' Not yesterday or tomorrow, but today. We need to learn to live one day at a time. We cannot rest if we are continuously dwelling on the past or worrying about the future.

"Another important way to ensure that you get enough rest is to make one day out of every seven a day of rest. A day to forget about the troubles at the office or mounting bills or social concerns. Make one day in every seven a day for you to enjoy with your family, to unwind the accumulated tension and relax.

"Just one day of rest every week seems so simple, I know, but it really is very important. All the major religions of the world refer to a sabbath, a day of rest. Perhaps God gave us a sabbath day to remind us that we need time to stop, to contemplate and relax. A sanctuary where we can be at peace with ourselves and the world."

The young man thought again about his life. Each day had its chores. He worked hard during the week and he was equally busy at the weekend. He often took work home with him. No wonder he had always felt so tired.

"Another very important and easy way to help you relax is deep breathing," explained Mr. Shaw.

"Oh yes, I met a wonderful lady who taught me how to do deep breathing exercises," the young man interjected. "Deep breathing helps clean the lymphatic system and nourish the body tissues."

"Yes it does, but it also helps relax the mind and body," said the businessman. "You see, when you get stressed and tense, your chest muscles tighten and this, of course, leads to various health problems. Deep breathing helps relax the chest and calms the nervous system. People who are very tense are usually very shallow breathers, whereas those people who are calm and relaxed breathe deeply.

"These are the fundamental principles of rest and believe me they changed my life completely. It is incredible when I think how my life was saved and turned around by a heart attack and a chance meeting in a train with an old Chinese man who made me aware of the importance of rest and relaxation."

When the young man got home later that evening he read over his notes from his extraordinary meeting.

The sixth secret of Abundant Health—the power of rest and relaxation. Abundant Health cannot be attained without resting the body and mind.

Rest:

- rejuvenates your mind, body, and spirit
- is vital to our physical and emotional health

- reduces the amount of oxygen our body requires by as much as 50 percent
- reduces the workload of the heart by as much as 30 percent
- lowers high blood pressure
- improves short and long term memory.

Take regular short breaks during the day.
Use the two-step formula to stop worrying.
Make one day in each week a day of rest.
Do deep breathing exercises especially when you are feeling stressed or nervous.

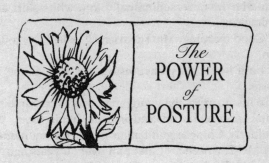

The
POWER
of
POSTURE

The seventh person on the young man's list was a man by the name of Ian Townsend. Mr. Townsend was a dentist who lived and worked at his home on the outskirts of the town. The young man was more than a little apprehensive about meeting Mr. Townsend, as he had never been at ease visiting dentists. He was also mystified as to what a dentist might have to say about Abundant Health.

The appointment had been made for 10 A.M. on Saturday and, as usual, the young man arrived bang on time with his trusted notepad in his hand and, on this occasion, his teeth very thoroughly brushed!

The young man was met by a small unassuming

man who was dressed casually in a white shirt and denim jeans.

"Good morning. Mr. Townsend?" asked the young man.

"I am he. It's a pleasure to meet you. Come in, please."

To his surprise, the young man was led not into the dental surgery, but instead into the living room. "So an elderly Chinese gentleman gave you my name," said Mr. Townsend. "I met him over 10 years ago . . . but when I close my eyes, I can still see him and hear his voice.

"I was very depressed and going through a difficult time. My physical health was deteriorating as well. I had recurrent bronchitis and terrible indigestion. All the hospital tests were negative, they couldn't find anything wrong with me, but I knew there had to be something causing my symptoms. If there was nothing wrong with me, as my doctor insisted, I wouldn't have been feeling so dreadful all the time.

"I really didn't want to take drugs to control my moods but I was getting desperate. Then, on a cold and dark morning, just before Christmas, I met your friend, the old man . . . and my life changed."

The young man sat spellbound, as Mr. Townsend related his story.

"I was walking my dog in the park as I always do. The grass was covered in frost, the day was only just beginning to dawn and I remember a full moon was still visible in the sky.

"I was throwing sticks for my dog to fetch when I suddenly had a severe coughing fit. It was so intense, and extremely painful. The next thing I remember was a hand on my shoulder and a gentle Asian voice telling me to sit down. I saw him then, an elderly Chinese man standing beside me, and I felt a warmth—actually it was more than warmth, it was heat—from his hand on my shoulder, and almost instantaneously, I stopped coughing.

"We both sat down on the park bench and talked for a few moments. It was then that I first heard about the secrets of Abundant Health. Needless to say, there were several important changes that I had to make in my life to improve my health, but there was one thing that was particularly relevant in my case, it was something I had never even considered before . . . the power of posture!"

"What do you mean?" asked the bewildered young man as he straightened himself in his chair.

"Well, as a dentist, I am continually hunched over people and, over the years, I developed rounded shoulders and an arched back. It happens to many people these days. Many professions, particularly sedentary office jobs, can cause bad posture. People are also developing poor posture from bad habits in childhood. Do you know that in western countries children spend an average of five hours every day sitting in front of the television, not to mention the amount of time they spend sitting playing computer games. The human body was not designed to live a sedentary lifestyle. Your posture—the way you stand, the way you sit, the way you walk, the way you hold yourself—is crucial to your health."

"But why is posture so important?" asked the perplexed young man.

"It's quite simple; in order for the tissues and organs to function properly and be healthy, they need two things—good blood supply and good nerve supply. The blood carries nutrients and oxygen to nourish and cleanse tissues and the nerve supply is like the electrical spark needed for energy. Without either of these, tissues will degenerate, waste away. What controls blood and nerve supply traveling through the body? Your posture!

"Imagine a garden hose: what happens when you pinch it?"

"The water stops flowing," answered the young man.

"Precisely. The same thing happens to the blood vessels and nerve pathways in our body; if they are pinched by displaced joints or muscle spasms, the blood circulation and nerve supply are hindered."

Mr. Townsend could tell by the look on the young man's face that he was still confused.

"Imagine your spine," continued the dentist. "You have 26 vertebrae and in between each one are blood vessels and nerve roots from the spinal cord. These feed the rest of your body. When you slouch, or sit awkwardly, the vertebrae pinch the blood vessels and nerve roots and in just the same way as water stops flowing when a garden hose is pinched, we literally starve our organs and tissues of blood and nerve energy when we have poor posture.

"Poor posture therefore leads to poor health; chest muscles become weak, leading to bronchitis and other respiratory problems—which is of course what happened to me—tummy muscles weaken and, as a result, the abdominal organs start to underfunction and often lead to a host of digestive disorders. Many people have this problem—a saggy tummy—and try to get rid of it by dieting. Whilst they may lose weight, they will always have a saggy tummy. No amount of dieting will get rid of a flabby tummy if you have poor posture."

"So a lot of people would do better to improve their posture to flatten their tummies rather than go on starvation diets?" said the young man.

"Absolutely. But posture does far more than just help flatten your stomach. Posture is the key to energy. The abdomen is considered by all ancient systems of medicine to be the energy center of the body. In Chinese medicine it is called the Chi, in the Indian Ayurvedic medicine, it is called the Hara. If the abdomen is weak, the energy center is weak and consequently we feel tired and listless."

The young man wrote notes as the dentist continued, "And one of the lesser-known facts about our posture is that it actually influences our emotions."

"How is that possible?" asked the young man.

"The way we hold ourselves actually influences our moods. Have you ever seen a depressed person standing erect, chest out, breathing deeply and smiling?"

The young man shook his head.

"And do you know why?" continued Mr. Townsend. "It is because our brain is stimulated by our posture. When we are depressed, we automatically slouch and drop our shoulders, and we tend to look down rather than straight ahead or up. The interesting thing is that once we are aware of this connection, we can more easily control our emotions and overcome depressive states just by changing our posture.

"You see, whilst you are standing or sitting erect, head held high, breathing deeply and smiling—even if you have no reason to smile—it is virtually impossible to become depressed."

"But surely it can't be that simple?" insisted the young man. "Depression is a complex emotional state."

"I'm not saying that correcting your posture is the only answer to depression. There are, after all, other factors such as negative attitudes, lack of faith, and suppressed emotions which all need to be considered and counseling may be necessary. But I am saying that we can all change our emotional states from negative to positive, we can all get out of a depressed state simply by changing our posture.

"Don't take my word for it, try it for yourself," urged the dentist. "Sit up straight, tuck your chin in, and imagine your head is being lifted up. Breathe deeply and smile."

The young man was embarrassed, but followed nonetheless and to his surprise, he immediately began to feel more energy and even more powerful. It was so simple, it made sense and, most important of all, it seemed to work!

"If a depressed state leads to poor posture," asked the young man, "does that mean that a happy disposition helps create better posture?"

"Naturally. Haven't you noticed how optimistic and happy people seem to hold their heads up in stark contrast to sad and depressed people whose heads are hung low and look down most of the time?"

"This is amazing," said the young man, gripped by the simplicity of what he was hearing. "But how do you improve your posture?"

"Well there are several easy ways to train your body to stay in its correct posture. Remember, your body instinctively 'knows' what its correct posture should be, the only thing is that it has learned bad habits.

"The first and most important point is *awareness*. Once you are aware of the importance of posture you will automatically be conscious of the way you hold yourself. This is why the first time I mentioned the word 'posture' to you earlier, you automatically sat upright!

"However, a healthy posture is never forced. Many people think they should stand to attention like a soldier—chest out, stomach pulled in—but this is not necessary. You should hold your head upright with your shoulders relaxed, hips slightly forward, and knees slightly bent, not locked.

"The secret to developing a healthy posture begins with awareness. We need to take time during the day to notice and become aware of the way we stand or sit, or even walk. Start to notice your postural habits, for example, the way you stand or sit at work, the way you sit at home when watching television, the way you stand when waiting in a queue. If you find, at times, that you are slouched, hunched over, and tense, take long, deep breaths and imagine that you are being gently pulled or stretched upward.

"Don't forget that we are all different. We have different-sized legs, torsos, arms. We have different

centers of gravity and consequently the best posture for one person may not be the best for another.
But we can all re-learn the best posture for our
bodies."

"How?" asked the young man.

"It is important to be aware of and correct any
bad habits. For instance, many secretaries and office
workers distort the posture of their upper back and
neck by holding the telephone between their neck
and ear. The muscles on one side become stronger
than the other side and pull the vertebrae out of
position."

The young man swallowed hard as he knew that
he often held his telephone in this way.

The dentist continued, "Parents who always lift
their child in the same arm and salesmen who always
carry their briefcase in the same arm are also damaging their posture. Boys delivering papers in the morn-
ings also often carry the heavy paper sack on the
same shoulder, day after day. It is particularly bad
when children's postures become distorted because
their bones are growing and this can lead to lifelong
postural problems.

"Some sports are one-sided and distort our postures. Tennis is a good example. Every time a player
serves he bends and twists his back and if this is
done often enough, it will cause postural problems
because one side of the back will be stronger than the
other.

"You see, the secret of correct posture is balance.
Continual imbalanced movements will create
imbalance."

"But you're not suggesting that people shouldn't

play one-sided sports such as tennis or golf, or that mothers shouldn't carry their babies, and you can't stop salesmen carrying heavy cases?" asked the young man.

"Of course not. I play tennis regularly myself," the dentist assured him, "and I am a parent too, but if we choose to play certain sports or if we have to do imbalanced things, we must correct the imbalance."

"How do you do that?"

"Well, it's very simple. Our joints are held in place by the soft tissues—the muscles, tendons, and ligaments. If the muscles on one side of a joint become stronger than the muscles on the other side, the joint is pulled out of its correct place and we have imbalanced posture. Therefore, if we do hold the phone between our neck and ear now and again, we should regularly stretch the neck the other way; if we play tennis regularly, before, during, and after the game we should twist and turn in the opposite direction to the way we serve or hit the ball; if we lift children or carry heavy briefcases regularly, we should use different sides alternately. It's really just common sense."

"Well, I can see that makes sense. Is there anything else which will help develop a healthy posture?" asked the young man.

"Yes, of course. Balanced exercise, a nutritious diet, and balanced emotions are also important. If muscles become weak from lack of exercise or poor nutrition, they will not be able to support the joints properly. Similarly, if we dwell on negative emotions, our posture will be affected. Although we can consciously control our posture, we cannot do so every minute of the day and in the long term the emotions will win over.

"Now I'm not saying that correcting your posture is the answer to all your problems because, as you know, there are 10 secrets of Abundant Health and they are all equally important. I'm also not suggesting that we should all go round every minute of each day sitting or standing erect and smiling—although I can't help imagining what a wonderful thing it would be if we did—but I am saying that once we are aware of the power of posture we can use it to improve our physical health and also to help control our emotional states as well."

At the end of the meeting, the young man thanked Mr. Townsend for his help and left. The dentist watched as the young man walked down the garden path with his head held high and he smiled to himself. There was a man who was beginning to use the power of his posture.

Later that day, the young man summarized the notes he had made.

The seventh secret of Abundant Health—the power of posture.

Good posture is vital to good health. Poor posture inhibits blood circulation, restricts nerve supply and leads to disease.

Our posture affects our moods and emotions as well as our physical health.

Good posture begins with awareness. Take time

every day to notice your posture and correct any bad postural habits.

Breathing deeply and imagining you are being gently pulled or stretched upward helps create a healthy posture.

The secret of good posture is "balance."

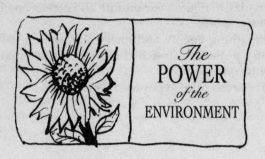

The POWER *of the* ENVIRONMENT

Peter Seagrove was a 45-year-old landscape gardener and lived in a small cottage on the outskirts of town. His was the eighth name on the young man's list and the young man was particularly curious to meet him.

"After all," the young man thought to himself, "what could a landscape gardener know about health?"

When the young man arrived he was met by a short man with a fresh, tanned complexion. Mr. Seagrove greeted the young man and shook his hand warmly.

"It's such a lovely day. Do you mind if we sit out back?" he asked.

"No, not at all. It's nice to be in the fresh air for a change," said the young man.

Mr. Seagrove led his guest along the garden path to the rear of the cottage, stopping occasionally to explain some of the plants and herbs he was growing. They arrived at a large pine table on a covered veranda and sat down. Mr. Seagrove poured them both some fresh apple juice and turned to the young man. "So what is it exactly you wish to know?" he asked.

The young man recounted his story and meeting with the old Chinese man.

"I see," said Mr. Seagrove.

"Who is the old man?" the young man asked.

"I don't know," said the gardener. "I met him once, 15 years ago. I was a different man in those days. Pale and weak, I suffered with chronic eczema and depression. I was really in a terrible state.

"Then one day I had a crisis which changed my life. It was a day when I was feeling particularly ill, so much so that I had to leave work early to go home. I got in the elevator and pressed the button for the ground floor. The elevator stopped a few floors down and a little old Chinese gentleman got in. The doors closed behind him and the lift continued its way down when it suddenly stopped between floors and the lights went out. The last time the lift broke down it had taken three hours before the repair men got it working again and so you can imagine how annoyed I was. I got more and more agitated, my head was pounding and felt as if it was going to explode.

"I said nothing, but in the darkness the old man said, 'Don't worry, it will be all right.' Before I could ask him what he meant, he said, 'Let me help you,' and I felt his hand touch the back of my neck. There was a sharp pain for an instant and then my headache was gone, totally gone. He had released something, like pulling a plug to let the water flow freely. I really couldn't believe it, it was like a miracle.

"I asked the old man what he had done to relieve the pain and he said he had used an ancient technique to release the electromagnetic tension in my neck which had been causing my headache. Well, as you can imagine, I was dumbfounded. How on earth did he know I had had a headache? And what was electromagnetic tension?

"He explained to me that radiation from office equipment—computers, photocopiers, faxes, VDU screens—all distort the magnetic fields and interfere with our health. He went on to talk about the secrets of Abundant Health. It was the first time I had heard that such simple things in our lifestyle could have such a dramatic effect on our health."

The young man could relate to that. He also had never imagined that his thoughts, his food, his posture, or any of the other secrets of Abundant Health could have had such a profound effect on his health. Yet, day by day, he was experiencing real changes.

"The old man gave me a list of people who would help me and they all did. Yet the one law that seemed to help me most was the Law of a Healthy Environment."

"What do you mean?" enquired the young man.

"Abundant Health cannot be created in an unhealthy environment. You see, people are simply not designed to work with no fresh air, no natural sunlight, and with high levels of radiation. Part of the reason for my illness had been my office. It made sense; after all, the workplace is where we spend most of our life.

"My office was fully equipped with the latest technology—computer terminals, VDUs, artificial lighting and air conditioning systems. These things create high levels of radiation and produce a very unhealthy, unnatural working environment.

"You see, I became aware of things so simple that most people never consider them. Things that are right in front of our noses but we do not see them. If we desire health we must create a healthy environment. We must ensure that the places in which we work, sleep, and live are conducive to health. You see, it is an established fact that the human body needs certain conditions just to survive, let alone to live.

"Let's take fresh air for starters. We can live for weeks without food and days without water, but not more than three minutes without oxygen. Yet so many people work in offices and factories that are air-conditioned. Stale air recycled day after day. How can this be healthy? We need to open the windows in our offices and in our bedrooms to get fresh oxygen in our lungs."

The young man recalled his visit to Mrs. Croft who had taught him the importance of deep breathing. "Without breath, there is no life," she had said. He realized that one could just as well say, "Without oxygen, there is no life." It was all making much more sense to him now. Like a jigsaw puzzle which, piece by piece, he was slowly putting together in his mind.

"What do you do if your office is situated on a

busy road? By opening the windows you might just be breathing in smog and dirt?" he asked Mr. Seagrove.

"There are only three choices—move jobs, ask your employer to get an air purifier, or accept the situation and breathe stale, polluted air."

Mr. Seagrove continued, "Then, of course, there is the question of daylight. Even if you are fortunate enough to work near a window in an office, more often than not it's tinted, blocking out natural daylight."

"But why is daylight so important?" asked the young man. "I thought the sun causes cancer."

"First of all, everything in this world if taken in excess can cause cancer or some other form of degenerative disease. It is true that if you expose your skin to excessive amounts of strong sunshine, it will burn and cause it to age and perhaps even lead to skin cancer. It is also true that this is becoming more of a problem now that the ozone layer is being eroded, which is another result of people neglecting their environment. A thinner ozone layer means less natural protection from the sun's rays and so people may burn more easily. But, the fact remains that we all need daylight, not necessarily direct strong sunshine, but exposure to ultraviolet rays.

"You see, every life form on this planet needs sunlight to survive. Man is no exception. Without daylight your body cannot produce vitamin D and without vitamin D you cannot metabolize calcium to produce bones and teeth. Without daylight your pineal gland, which is a small but very important gland in your head, cannot function. The pineal gland helps regulate blood sugar levels, hormones, and even our emotions, which is why many people suffer with Seasonal Affective Disorder."

"I have heard of Seasonal Affective Disorder," interrupted the young man, "but what is it exactly?"

"Seasonal Affective Disorder is a condition that is caused by lack of sunlight which can produce a multitude of health complaints including chronic fatigue, anxiety, depression, weight gain, rheumatic pains, sadness, and even low sexual drive. It occurs primarily in the winter and for the most part disappears in the spring. It is now possible to bring daylight indoors by using special fluorescent lighting which approximates to the wavelengths of natural sunlight. Of course, natural sunlight is better."

"What about other environmental factors? You mentioned that you were affected by electromagnetic radiation."

"Yes. The radiation from computers, VDUs, laser printers, photocopiers, artificial strip lighting, and other electronic equipment often reaches levels which are hazardous to our health. There is increasing evidence linking radiation levels not just to migraines and skin problems like eczema, but also to leukemia and other cancers, and even to infertility."

The young man was alarmed. "What can be done about it?" he asked. "People can't just up and change their jobs."

"No, they can't. But, if you can't take your job to Nature, take Nature to your job. Open the windows, ask for better quality lighting, and bring lots of plants into your workplace."

"How do plants help?" enquired the young man.

"Common household plants are the best environmental purifiers. Tests conducted by NASA—the American space organization—have confirmed that common house plants remove most of the toxic gases and environmental pollutants by absorbing them through the leaves and roots. Plants also absorb and eliminate excessive radioactivity."

"That's incredible," said the young man. "So we can create a healthy environment simply by bringing plants into the workplace, getting more fresh air, and more natural sunlight."

"Precisely," said Mr. Seagrove. "You've got it in one. But more than our own working environment, we all need to be concerned about the world environment. After all, what hope is there for our children and grandchildren, if our generation bequeaths polluted waters, polluted land, and polluted air? We must realize that the future depends upon the present, we must act now to restore the balance in Nature and re-create a healthy environment the way Nature intended."

The young man had never realized that the condition of his immediate environment was so important to his health and he had certainly not contemplated the possibility that he could influence the environment in which he lived and worked. "Wouldn't it be something," he thought, "if everyone tried to improve their immediate environment—at work and at home—to create health now and ensure a healthier life for future generations?"

Later that evening the young man read through his notes.

The eighth secret of Abundant Health—abundant health cannot be created in an unhealthy environment.

Fresh, clean air and daylight are the cornerstone of a healthy environment.

If you can't take your work to Nature, take Nature to your work.

Take care of your immediate environment and play your part to restore balance and harmony in the environment throughout the world.

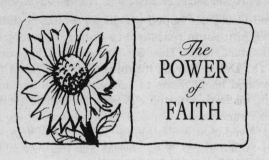

The
POWER
of
FAITH

The following night the young man was wakened by the sound of thunder and flashes of lightning. He got up and stood by his bedroom window looking out at the storm. Sometimes he had confused and troubled moments like this. Despite the progress he had made and lessons he had learned, sometimes it all seemed too unbelievable. There was no doubt that he was feeling better but was his body deceiving him? Earlier that day he had been told by a consultant physician at the hospital that his disease may have gone into remission. As a result, the young man was tormented by doubts and fears. What if the expert was right?

The young man's thoughts turned to the next

person on his list, a retired doctor by the name of Dr. Emil Dobre. He hoped the doctor would be able to give him some reassurance about the secrets of Abundant Health. The next day he would find out.

Dr. Dobre's gray, thinning hair and lined face revealed his 80 years of age, although it had to be said, his large, clear blue eyes had a certain youthful appearance about them. Dr. Dobre was obviously overjoyed to meet the young man and welcomed him with open arms. A few weeks ago the young man would have been embarrassed at the thought of being embraced by a total stranger, but somehow it felt safe and natural.

It was not long before they both sat down and the young man told the doctor of his worries.

Dr. Dobre leaned forward and said, "You do not need to worry. You are on the right path and so long as you stay on the path, you will get better. Remission is just a medical word that doctors sometimes use when a patient gets better without any medical interference. Many doctors do not understand the concept of Abundant Health and presume that our health is due to luck, but you and I know differently, don't we?" Dr. Dobre smiled to the young man.

"But the doctor who saw me yesterday was a specialist," insisted the young man.

"Ah, well that explains it," said Dr. Dobre. "Do you know what George Bernard Shaw said about specialists? He said a specialist is someone who knows more and more about less and less until he knows absolutely everything about nothing at all!"

They both laughed. The young man was beginning to feel a bit easier.

"The secrets of Abundant Health," said Dr. Dobre, "are like the stars—they are there for all to see but we must still look for them. Many people believe health comes with medicines and they look nowhere else. At medical school, I was taught that man was a machine which could be serviced like a car. I was taught that the key to health was new and better medications. I qualified as a doctor at the University of Prague in 1936 but it was during the Second World War that I learned my greatest lesson in medicine . . . the power of faith."

"What do you mean?" asked the young man, somewhat perplexed.

"Man is not just a machine, we are not just flesh and bones. We have spirit, an essence which is more than chemicals and molecules. We all have a spirit that can rise above the limitations of the body."

The young man listened intently as the doctor continued.

"During the war, I spent four years in a German concentration camp surviving on meager rations of stale bread with a cup of warm water they described as soup. There was no nourishment to speak of—no vitamins, no protein, no real nutrients, and even today, scientists cannot understand how people survived for so long, living on so little."

"How did you survive?" asked the young man.

"I attribute my survival to one thing—faith! I had dysentery near the end of the war. I couldn't eat anything and I was losing a lot of blood. The pain was so terrible that I finally collapsed and felt that death would be a welcome relief. All I could do was pray . . . "

Tears began to well up in the doctor's eyes. "It was then that your friend came," he whispered. "In the middle of the night an old Chinese man knelt down beside me and held my hand. I can still hear the echo of his voice. 'Have faith, my friend,' he said. 'You will not die, have faith.' He stayed with me throughout the night but when I awoke the next day he was gone. Though my body was wasting, my spirit clung on to the old man's promise of life and the next day the war ended and the camp was liberated. I was carried out on a stretcher weighing less than 40 kilos. But . . . " Dr. Dobre was struggling to whisper the words, "the old oriental man was right . . . I was alive."

The young man swallowed hard. It was difficult to imagine the tall man before him weighing so little.

The doctor continued, "The old Chinese man saved my life and he taught me the most valuable lesson I have ever learned in medicine."

"What was that?" asked the young man.

"Where there is faith, there is life."

"But what do you mean by 'faith'?" enquired the young man.

"Faith, it is written, is the substance of things hoped for, the evidence of which remains unseen. Faith is a spiritual conviction, a belief in things which cannot be validated by the five senses. Faith is a spiritual power with which the impossible becomes possible. It is the solution to all problems, the hope in all despair, the light at the end of all tunnels. Faith is the force which can move mountains."

"But faith in what?" persisted the young man.

"Faith in life, faith in yourself, and faith in a Higher Power," answered the doctor. "Of course, many in my profession would call this nonsense but they refuse to look upward and so they never see the stars."

"But couldn't the power of your mind have had something to do with your recovery?" asked the young man. "I learned recently that you can use your mind to heal your body, and *believing* that you will recover can often in itself bring about the recovery."

"That is very true," answered Dr. Dobre, "but faith connects the human spirit to a higher power, stronger even than the power of the mind. Let me ask you something; do you believe in God? By that I mean a Creator of life or a Higher Intelligence."

"I am not sure."

"Well, let me show you something." And the doctor led the young man into another room. In the corner was a large object nearly two meters tall, covered by a sheet. The doctor walked up to it and pulled the sheet away. "Da-da!" he exclaimed as he exposed a clockwork planetarium. He wound the key and all the planets in the earth's solar system moved in their orbits around the sun.

The young man was aghast with awe, mesmerized by the perfect timing and movement of the planets. "Where did you get this?" he asked.

"Oh, it just formed itself," smiled Dr. Dobre. "Over the past 10 years the pieces have formed themselves into what you see before you."

"No. Come on, be serious," persisted the young man. "Where did you get it?"

"I tell you it evolved by itself," answered the doctor.

"Now anyone can see that this machine must have been made by someone," argued the young man.

"Ah ha! Now listen to yourself. You insist that this clockwork model has been created. Yet this is a poor imitation of the real thing.

"Our solar system is infinitely more complex, the timing of the whole universe needs no mechanism, yet each star has always maintained its own orbit. You see, to suggest that the universe and the life within it has evolved or to think that mankind developed from amoeba over thousands of years is far more ridiculous than saying this clockwork planetarium put itself together. It's like saying that the *Oxford Dictionary* was formed by an explosion in a print factory. Do you see? Where there is design, there must also be a designer."

"Yes, I do."

"To me, faith in a God or a Higher Power—it really doesn't matter what name we choose to give it—but faith in a power greater than ourselves, is essential to our well-being. It is written, 'Man does not live by bread alone but by every word that proceeds out of the living God.'"

"It sounds nice, but what does it mean?" asked the young man.

"That we need more than just physical nourishment, we need spiritual nourishment as well."

"But surely you are not suggesting that to be healthy one must believe in God. There are many people I know who are atheists who are perfectly healthy."

"Of course, you can survive, you can live and get by without believing in God, but there is rarely any long lasting fulfilment and Abundant Health without it.

"My experiences as a doctor have left me with no doubt whatsoever that faith is one of the most important factors in healing. And I am not alone in this view. Professor Claude E. Forkner, former President of the New York Cancer Society, once said: 'Very often we do not know what it is that brings about the recovery of the patient. I am sure that often it is faith which is a most important factor,' and Dr. Elmer Hess, MD, wrote: 'A physician who walks into a sickroom is not alone. He can only minister to the ailing person with the material tools of scientific medicine—his faith in God does the rest.'

"You see, faith creates trust, peace of mind. It releases a force that can perform miracles. Faith has been shown to be a vital factor in people recovering from supposedly 'incurable' diseases, therefore it should also be considered an important part of creating Abundant Health.

"The opposite of faith," continued the doctor, "is doubt, fear, anxiety, and worry. All of which are health destroying. This is perhaps why those people who maintain a sincere faith not only are generally healthier than those who do not, but they also recuperate faster when they do fall ill.

"If your faith is strong enough, it can not only help you, but it will help others as well. It's not so strange when you think about it. All religious scriptures tell of healing through faith. In the Bible there is a story of the prophet Elijah healing a dying young boy and, of course, there are plenty of references to Jesus healing the sick with the power of his faith."

The young man thought about some of the people he had visited who said they had been saved by the old man just touching them. Now he understood, the old man had used the power of his own faith to help them.

"When all is said and done," said the doctor, "there is a power in this world much greater than men or machines. It is available to anyone, anywhere, and at anytime."

"Are you saying that faith will cure anything?"

"The power of faith is unlimited but of course, as it is written, 'Faith without action is worthless.' If we continue to live our lives contrary to the laws of Nature, all the faith in the world will not help us in the long run because nothing can escape the universal law of cause and effect."

"So, how do people find faith?" asked the young man. "I have had no religious upbringing to speak of."

"Oh, you don't have to be a member of any religious group to believe in a Higher Power. The Creator of the Universe is the Creator of everyone and everything in this world, not just a select group of people," said the doctor. "Remember, faith has nothing to do with religion, it is something inside you. To find it, all we need do is search. Sometimes we are fortunate and something occurs to show us the way."

"What sort of thing?" said the young man.

"Well, perhaps a crisis!" said the doctor. "A crisis is like the storm at night, it can disperse the clouds of confusion, and clear the sky. And afterward, if you look up, you might see the stars."

The doctor continued, "For years I was convinced that the old Chinese man was a figment of my dreams. Not one other camp survivor saw him and I had never seen him before nor have I seen him since. But then, more than a year later, I had confirmation that he was most definitely real."

"What happened?" asked the young man.

"Someone just like you knocked on my door," smiled the doctor.

That night the young man lay awake in bed writing notes about his meeting with Dr. Dobre.

> *The ninth secret of Abundant Health—the power of faith.*

Faith is the spiritual power with which the impossible becomes possible.

Faith connects the human spirit with a Higher Power.

To attain Abundant Health, we need more than physical nourishment, we need spiritual nourishment as well.

Faith releases a force which can perform miracles.

The opposite of faith is worry, doubt, fear, and anxiety.

Faith without action is worthless.

A howling wind whistled outside and the rain thrashed against the bedroom window. In time, the storm passed, leaving a peaceful silence. The young man got up, went to the window, and looked up. "Well, what do you know?" he said softly to himself. The night sky was alight, filled with an ocean of glittering stars. At that moment, all his doubts and all his fears and all his worries began to fade.

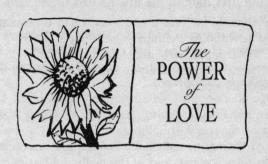

The
POWER
of
LOVE

Forty days had passed since the young man had begun his quest and during that short period of time he had not only learned about Abundant Health but he had also put that knowledge into practice.

He had spent time each day doing healing visualizations and affirmations, he had practiced deep breathing exercises and made sure he did some form of physical exercise every day. He had changed his diet, and he had become more conscious of his posture; he made a special effort to look out for things that made him smile and laugh, and he brought plenty of big green plants into his home and office to create a healthier living environment. He had rested, physically and mentally, and for the first time in his life, he had found faith in himself and in life.

The young man had been living by the laws of Abundant Health and had never felt better. To his amazement and delight, his original symptoms had completely disappeared.

He was not sure what more he could learn, but there remained one more name on his list. It was a lady by the name of Edith James. And so it was with mixed feelings of anticipation and apprehension that he knocked on the door of the tenth and last person on his list.

Mrs. James was an elderly lady with rosy cheeks and smiling eyes. She had an almost tangible warmth, a glow surrounding her which reminded the young man of the old Chinese man. He knew instantly that Mrs. James was obviously a very special person.

"I must say, this is a wonderful surprise," she said to the young man. "From what you told me over the phone, you must have met Dr. Dow."

"I didn't know that was his name?"

"Well, I really don't know for sure either, but it's the name I have given him."

"Why? What's the significance?" asked the young man.

"Well, 'Dow' is actually spelled T-A-O. It is Chinese for 'way' or 'path.' I gave him that name because he guided me on a path back to health. It was well over 50 years ago but I remember it as if it were yesterday. I had a very dangerous illness— tuberculosis—but I had no idea how serious it was until I overheard a doctor talking to a nurse outside my ward. He asked her to check up on me every two hours. When the nurse asked why, he gave her a reply which I will never forget. He told her to give me whatever food I wanted because I had less than a month to live!

"As you might imagine, I was totally devastated. I wasn't ready to die. I was only 23 years old. After the initial shock, I spent the rest of the day with my eyes firmly shut, praying. In the evening, an old Chinese man knocked on my door offering magazines to read. I was in no mood to read but he gave me such a warm smile and said he had brought a special magazine just for me. So I took it.

"He stayed for a few moments and we talked about life, and the subject quickly turned to health. It was then I first heard of the secrets of Abundant Health and the old man gave me a list of people who, he said, would help me. I couldn't stop myself bursting into tears because I knew I was dying. The old man came over and put his arms around me, and said everything was going to be fine. The last thing I heard him say: 'There is a special message for you in the magazine. Please read it.'

"After he had left and I had stopped sobbing and dried my eyes, I picked up the magazine and started to read. It was just as well that I did, because it really did contain a very special message for me which saved my life."

The young man sat and listened, spellbound.

"You might ask what sort of article could save a young, dying woman," Mrs. James continued. "It was not about health or medicine, just a simple story. But to me it was no ordinary story because it seemed to be telling my father's life.

"My parents divorced when I was just five years old and I never heard of or saw my father much afterward. He was a prominent architect and I had always assumed that he never cared for me; my mother and I moved away and I never once received so much as a birthday card from him. But the truth came out in the magazine when it described a frustrated architect, born in my father's hometown, who went to my father's school and university and then married a beautiful blonde Austrian lady 15 years his junior. An architect who left a bitterly unhappy marriage and was denied seeing his only daughter. It had to be him. The story told how he wrote many letters to his daughter and always sent birthday and Christmas gifts, but not once did he receive a reply or even an acknowledgment, and after 14 years he gave up and found comfort in a new marriage and a new family.

"All my life I had felt unloved by my father and all the time he had felt unloved by me. The truth of course was that my mother's anger and bitterness led her to hide all his letters and gifts. She made me want to hate my father for all those years. Now, on my deathbed, I knew for the first time in my life that I was loved and missed and cared for by my father. I was determined to let him know that I loved him too before I died.

"When I finished reading the story in the magazine I decided to telephone my father immediately. I didn't know his phone number or even his address but the article mentioned the town in which he lived, so it wasn't difficult to get his number. I hadn't spoken to him for nearly 20 years and when he answered the phone, I burst into tears.

"The very next morning my father was by my bed-side holding my hand. It was a strange feeling, difficult to explain, but I felt as if I had been given a miracle elixir. I regained my appetite and within a few days I was walking through the beautiful grounds of the hospice each day with my father. I savored the fresh mountain air and the scent of the rose garden.

"The doctors had been monitoring me during this time and took various samples to check on the progress of the disease. Then one day, whilst my father and I were sitting in the rose garden, a doctor came running out of the building shouting to me and waving some papers. The tests this time were all negative. Would you believe it, there were no signs whatsoever of tuberculosis. I was going to live after all!"

"That must have been an incredible feeling," said the young man.

"Oh, believe me, it was. Yet it was later that evening that I realized that I had never really thanked the old Chinese man who brought me the magazine or told him how the magazine had helped reunite me with my father. So I went to the hospital personnel department and asked if they could put me in touch with the old Chinese man who had worked on my ward and handed out magazines. But . . ."

"Don't tell me," interrupted the young man, "they had no records of a Chinese man on their staff."

Mrs. James smiled. "Of course."

"Why do you think you made such a dramatic recovery?" asked the young man, changing the subject.

"Well, as you might expect, the doctors were completely mystified. I think my recovery was probably due to a combination of factors—diet; fresh, clean mountain air; prayer and exercise. I learned the importance of them after I left hospital from the people on the old man's list. But there is no doubt in my mind that the biggest breakthrough in my health was brought about through something rarely spoken of in medicine or healing and that is . . . the power of love.

"I know it sounds rather odd but I assure you it is true."

"Really?" said the young man. "Love helped cure your tuberculosis?"

"Most definitely. Love is spoken of in all ancient scriptures as the strongest force in the universe—love has the power to conquer all!

"I once read a wonderful, true story of a certain traveler in the cold, snowy prairies in North America which illustrates the power of love. On one of his travels in the middle of winter the traveler became lost in a snowstorm between two mountain villages. Exhausted and frozen he could travel no further and he lay down to die. But barely a moment later he heard a child crying. He stumbled toward the child, groping in the blizzard, and found a little girl lying in the snow. He picked the girl up and held her tight to his chest to keep her as warm as he could and he marched on, determined to save the little girl's life. No more than 100 paces further was a lone log cabin. It was the little girl's home. The traveler had saved her life and in so doing had saved his own.

"This is true love, unconditional love, helping without regard for profit because the reward is in the doing. In helping others, we help ourselves. There are many laws in the universe, all of them precise and unfailing, but the greatest of them all is the Law of Love because Love outlives everything, it is the strongest force in the universe. With love, we can overcome all adversity, all problems . . . and all sickness. I firmly believe that "love" is often an important element which helps overcome many diseases and is all too often neglected. And I have no doubt whatsoever that without abundant love we can never find Abundant Health."

"But why is love so important for our health?" asked the young man.

"Love is important to health because it is an essence of life. Without it life loses purpose and meaning and ultimately we become depressed. The opposite of love—hate, selfishness, anger, and resentment—all create poisons in the body which will kill us as surely as the most toxic of chemicals.

"Love nourishes our mind, body, and spirit. In fact, it has been shown that people who feel loved recover much faster from illness than people who feel unloved."

"How is that?" asked the young man.

"Well, when we feel loved, the number of our white blood cells increases, special hormones are released in the body to help us cope with stress and pain, and the whole disposition of a patient becomes totally transformed. A few years ago an interesting study was done at a London teaching hospital which actually proved how love promotes healing. The surgeon normally would go round the ward visiting patients the night before their operation to explain the nature of their operation. On this occasion, though, the surgeon held his patients' hands and was generally more caring as he talked with them. Defying all clinical explanation, these patients recovered, on average, three times faster than the other patients!

"Love is a crucial element not only in overcoming disease but also in maintaining health. Many people become sick because they do not love themselves. They feel unloved and unhappy and, many times, they have difficulties in their personal relationships. But love is available to everyone. There is one way in which we can be guaranteed to receive love."

"What is it?" asked the young man.

"We always receive love . . . when we give love."

"I think I know what you mean," said the young man. "Whenever I help someone or make them smile, I feel great."

"Exactly," said Mrs. James, "and the more we give, the more we get back. And the more we love, the better we feel. It's quite wonderful, isn't it?"

Mrs. James handed the young man a plaque. "This says it all for me. It is a passage written by a man called Emmett Fox in his book entitled *Sermon on the Mount*."

On the plaque were inscribed the following words:

> There is no difficulty that enough love will not conquer; no disease that enough love will not heal; no door that enough love will not open; no gulf that enough love will not bridge; no wall that enough love will not throw down; no sin that enough love will not redeem . . .
> It makes no difference how deep seated may

be the trouble; how hopeless the outlook . . . a sufficient realization of love will dissolve it all. If only you could love enough you would be the happiest and most powerful being in the world . . .

Later that day the young man read over the brief notes he had made.

The tenth secret of Abundant Health—the power of love

Love is the eternal healing force.
The secret in receiving love lies in giving it.

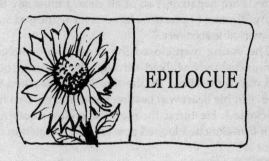

EPILOGUE

Five years later the young man was older and wiser. He had become a writer and lecturer in natural health care, passing on the knowledge that had changed his life. He taught by his own example, living every day with respect for the laws of Abundant Health.

He remembered the day he had gone back to his doctor exactly 10 weeks after his first visit. It was an anxious moment, more nerve-wracking than his original visit 10 weeks earlier. The doctor sat before him silently reading through the results of the recent tests. Two minutes passed but, to the young man, it seemed like hours. Finally, the doctor removed his spectacles and looked up at the young man.

"Well," he said, smiling, "I'm delighted to say that

all tests are negative. You're all clear. I must say that in my 30 years of practice I have never witnessed such a remarkable recovery."

The young man closed the surgery door behind him and slowly walked through the waiting room and out of the clinic. By the time he had reached the main exit his heart was beating faster and his step had quickened. He burst through the swing doors and with fists clenched looked upward and shouted in full voice . . .

"YES!"

The secrets of Abundant Health had led the young man out of the despair of ill health and into the joy of Abundant Health. Yet not a day went by when the young man did not think of the little old Chinese man who helped change the course of his life. He now understood what a precious gift his original illness had been because it had led him to a richer, more fulfilled life. He wished he could let the old man know what had happened as a result of their meeting. He wished he could tell him that he now understood what the old man had meant and thank him for his help.

Suddenly his thoughts were interrupted by the ringing of the telephone. It was a woman who asked if she could meet with him. She had been told he would be able to help her. Could she see him as soon as possible?

"Certainly. How would tomorrow afternoon suit you? Say, 3 P.M.?"

"That would be wonderful. Thank you so much," exclaimed the woman. "I am very grateful. I was told you will know exactly how to help me."

"I'll do my best," he assured her. "But tell me, who was it that gave you my number?"

"I'm afraid I don't know his name. I only met him this morning. He said he was a friend of yours . . . an elderly Chinese man."

The young man smiled to himself as he put down the phone and in a soft whisper said, "God bless you, Dr. Tao, wherever you are."

Adam J. Jackson is an internationally renowned therapist, author, and motivational speaker. He originally practiced law in England before retraining in natural health sciences. He currently lives in the United Kingdom and heads health clinics both there and in Toronto, Canada.

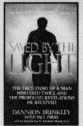
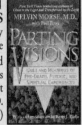

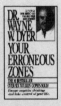
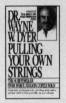